I0479838

Winter Flowers

Inspiring Stories of Recovery

James David Michell

Forward

Winter Flowers: Blooming During Struggles

Approximately 90 million Americans have some type of a mental illness, while less than half of them seek treatment. There are many reasons treatment is not sought, stigma and fear being among the top of those reasons. The other half of Americans that do receive treatment are either handling their illness through private means with insurance in hand, while yet another part of this population of people are inundated into what is referred to by many as the system. That system is the mental health system which is there with a clinic as its base offering doctor care and supposed psychosocial rehabilitation. I use the term 'supposed' due to the fact that psychosocial rehabilitation has very little time afforded to it because much of the case worker's time it devoted to every day needs such as taking consumers to doctor's appointments, medication checks, and other basic needs of the consumers.

The book in which I have written contains a twofold purpose. One is to hopefully get it out to those who are in that system and that it made be used successfully to incorporate a non linear approach to the care my peers receive. I am a consumer myself, and also a peer provider where I have worked as a QMHP on the ACT team and other various positions throughout my 15 year tenure as a consumer of services. The other goal of this book is that it would be there made readily available to the person who suffers in silence and alone, fearful and unwilling to incorporate into their lives the different organizations which provide support and help for the fear of being labeled by society.

The recovery workbook is drafted into four phases. The simplicity in which it denotes itself is that each phase builds upon the previous where in the completion of the workbook, the consumer hopefully finds, through their own, incorporation of knowledge gained and practices done, the recovery which is sought out by them and one which they see fruitful in their own eyes.

I do believe in peer support practices and the empathetic nature which only it can bring to a consumer through the sharing of experiences and within this book are inspirational examples of that process. However, I also believe that a recovery program should be clinical as well. In this workbook the clinical applications along with practical usable skills are incorporated into one whole curriculum using both the strengths from each of the recovery ideas to bring about recovery.

I find that the main recovery stances which SAMSHA has put out in terms of the ten basic concepts of recovery useful and these are implanted throughout the course of the curriculum. I also find it interesting that we inn this profession of service workers enjoy playing with the alphabet when we indicate what type of service we provide, so here to it continues in the different phases with each of the letters in each of the four phases representing a critical aspect of recovery from the standpoints we examined earlier. The four phases are putting your recovery into MOTION, how to ACTIVATE your recovery, how to MANAGE your recovery and final how you BENEFIT from your recovery.

While the recovery workbook does have topics on doctors and medication, as well as symptom management, it is more of a holistic approach by which all of these topics which are useful in mastering during recovery form one of the four major mental illnesses, are also useful in everyday life interactions.

Finally this workbook was comprised as I decided to take on what I felt was lacking in the realm of peer support and that is there is no unified curriculum of which to go by. I have been a peer support facilitator and have attended workshops and the such, but always found my colleagues grasping on to the same old symptom management curriculum resulting in repetition and boredom for my peers and no further advancement in their journey of recovery. The outline of the workbook is each chapter will contain an article written about the recovery topic, followed by an inspirational portion where success in application of the topic is evaluated. Then a participation portion where the consumer is able to do more evaluation of other peers engagements, and work out for themselves out of what they have learned, a plan in order form them to follow and reflect on during the process of working their recovery.

My vision is to see this sold as a workbook faltering on the side of a self help book in the bookstores, and then for those in the system we examined a new basis of which to tackle to project of recovery. I also see the workbook as something tangible which can be, used and billed for the sake of insurances, But more importantly for the sake of the recovery of an individual from a debilitating disease.

Recovery I believe is a responsibility and one which I take on daily. Recovery is a responsibility to one's self, to their loved ones and society as a whole. It is my hope that all who read this book are inspired to gain a strong foothold on recovery, and the topics throughout will help with empowerment of and individual not only in the realm of their disease , but also spread and effect all ares of their life, making them a person with the feeling of wholeness, where the moments of life do not pass them by due to the twofold process we find ourselves as mental health consumers undertaking. That twofold role of consumer and any other roles which one might take on as a responsibility.

Introduction

We as consumers have been told many times which way we should recover and what it means to be recovered. There are some people in the field of mental health who don't believe that recovery is even possible. While we should be aware and work in tandem with the clinics and doctors who help us to achieve recovery, it is ultimately a responsibility which we must take on ourselves. In taking on that responsibility we should make sure to have the measurements of recovery determined by ourselves. Making recovery work for us means that it works in our lives, and is successful for us by the way we view it in our eyes. Finding the means and method by which to achieve that is an adventure on its own, as there are several ways in which to utilize recovery concepts. Gathered together in this book are many topics which focus on recovery, and promote the active involvement by the consumer as they create their own recovery plan. This book is written with clinical aspects as well as practiced and practical concepts developed through the eyes of a peer.

The format of this book is divided into four phases, starting with the phase of putting your recovery into motion. The second, third and fourth phases are aimed at activating your recovery, managing recovery and final benefiting from your efforts by participating in recovery.

As consumers we seek out a better way in which to function in life while eliminating the issues which come with having a mental illness. We should look at recovery as a responsibility for ourselves, our loved ones, and society as a whole. Perhaps the most important aspect of recovery is the continued engagement within practicing the concepts. We are a unique people of strengths whereby we have shown perseverance in our position as a people of resilience. Recovery is actual and factual and I hope that you find in this book the inspiration and means by which to find it for yourself.

Motion

The first phase of putting your recovery in to motion is a good place to start, as to begin something you must first start it by putting the process into motion. In this phase many concepts are looked at, geared towards making the transition into recovery one which is filled with a hope of a new beginning and inspiration as to where you are going as you create your own method of recovery.

Different concepts of possible roadblocks which are common to us as consumers and the ways by which we can overcome them are examined. The importance of knowing all about our diagnosis, and whether we agree with it or we do not, is a question worth investigating. Also the importance of using all that information gathered towards making your goal of recovery a reality.

The first topic in this motion phase of recovery is motivation. Motivation is important to any aspect in life that people undertake. For us as consumers it can be said that it is even more important, as we have a position or stance on which to start our recovery process, with the hope that the things that motivate us will come to fruition.

Chapter one

Motivation

Incorporating a daily affirmation, along with your everyday routine, is a good tool in recovery. One which I often use is: "WAKE UP, SELF. YOU ARE BEING PRODUCTIVE. YOU ARE ENGAGED IN RECOVERY."

These words have several positive, affirmative applications towards recovery. When you tell yourself to "wake up," you are clearing your mind of any negative thoughts and stressors that your mind may be occupied with at the time. Also, we, as consumers, often find ourselves in a daze from the effects of our medication, and this helps to give us a sense of being alert. Secondly, the need for human beings to be productive is innate. Being productive is judged in many facets of life. For us, as consumers, to be productive in our other roles, which we chose to maintain responsibility in, we must first apply ourselves to being productive in our role as consumers and the responsibility of being engaged in recovery.

We all are in the process of recovery; and by being in that process, it means that something acted as a motivator to begin that engagement process. It could be that our loved ones or support networks have seen us hurt and researched where to get the assistance we need. It may be that we ourselves were tired of fighting the symptoms of our illness and sought help independent of others. Whatever way we have come to the stage of recovery which we are in, there was a motivating factor behind our willingness to participate.

Now that we are here, engaging in this process of recovery, we should also be aware that our recovery is based on our own needs as individuals. We must explore and be aware of the needs which must be met in our own particular journey of recovery. It is essential for us to become aware of what motivated us to take on the responsibility of recovery. Without a purpose for our actions we are left without anything to pursue. This can lead us into idleness when dealing with life, and this idle state of being can damage our spirit, our self esteem, and our motivations. When this occurs, the symptoms of our illness can become agitated and prevent the dreams and aspirations, which we have in life, from evolving into a reality.

Learning to make application of our motivators or driving forces is an essential key to our success. These often tend to change as we reach different stages of recovery. Taking some looks at examples of motivators can be helpful. A couple of the common ones we tend to share are: wanting to feel better and having our symptoms alleviated. We should ask ourselves: "In what ways can I make that a reality?"

We can seek assistance in the management of symptoms from members of our therapeutic teams. We can make the choice to manage our medications. We can participate in peer support groups. We can education ourselves about our diagnoses and the coping strategies needed to manage our mood and thought disorders. These are all ways of applying motivation in recovery. Motivation is not only a thought which drives you, but also an action.

It is important to remember our motivations as we go forward in our recovery. It is helpful to gage each one as to how we have shown resiliency by what we have achieved along the way. This allows us to look back upon milestones and be proud of what we have done and achieved. This gives us an even greater sense of hope as to what we eventually want to achieve in our goals or aspirations, or roles that we wish to maintain or fulfill in life. There is nothing more exciting and fulfilling than being a participant in growth, and nothing more helpful than looking back on the history of that growth and examining the ways in which you achieved it. You can use that history as a guideline as to what did work in your recovery and use them again. You can see what activities acted as a stumbling block, and learn from those, so as to not to become stuck in a state of non worthwhile repetitiveness.

In looking back at my two episodes where I became so unable to handle my mental health that hospitalization was required, I remember the motivators that pushed me forward in my recovery. To one begin that recovery, and two to sustain it. The first was my initial psychiatric hospitalization where I was brought there, by ambulance, after being tended to at the emergency room by doctors who were busy with the job of sewing up the deep cuts that I made in my wrists, after a failed suicide attempt. I spent the week in the hospital there, listening to the group therapists, and abiding by taking my meds. But when I was on the outside of those locked doors of the hospital is where my motivation would be important. I would find that motivation which I needed at the time in the sense of success in a career.

I had been attending college for two years now, all while suffering silently with the disease of schizophrenia and its symptoms, and after my hospitalization felt the need to work, in the hope that worthwhile activity and being productive would get my mind off things. Working is beneficial to us as consumers as we gain a sense of accomplishment through it, amongst other things, like financial security, but for me I picked a position where I was career bound, again adding to the motivation reliance I had with hopes of being successful. So I rallied upon my past strengths of when I was in my teen years where I enjoyed the opportunity to work at different restaurants, and sought solace at an upper echelon country club which I was living near at the time. This brought much excitement with being active around the golf scene and tournaments coming through, and I enjoyed the hustle and bustle of the fast paced restaurant atmosphere.

While there, working long hours throughout the week, I did researching my off time about how to further my career in the industry. I learned of the different organizations to become a member which could help further your career in that field, and the colleges you could go to whose curriculum centered in around restaurant management. I was excited by the promotions that I was afforded there at the country club, and the intake of more responsibilities placed upon me, as I was learning firsthand knowledge though my employment. My motivation was centered around being successful in my career. This was an easy choice for a motivator for me, as it was brought about by how I saw myself as a failure. I was a past user of illicit drugs, and know what I referred to then as a mental health patient. I felt a need to find an avenue of success in my life, one which I could measure through the tasks I accomplished and the societal view of a worthy career. While this worked for a while, keeping busy and having my motivation being driven by hopeful success, I still did not realize that, to be completely successful in all of my life choices, I first needed to be successful in my recovery. But I was new to being a mental health consumer and information of being able to assess your phase in recovery, and act on the strengths gathered thus far, I did not know could assist you in all aspects. While this motivator came naturally, I did not proceed with further steps, where to concurrently work on my lifestyle expectations, as well as my recovery, and this too did eventually fall apart again under the demands of the job, and I had yet another setback, whereby the position was lost to me, and I delved further into what was now a progressive illness.

I then proceeded with looking for motivators to keep me engaged in my recovery, as the last time around I lost interest so much, due to disappointment in what I then saw as failure in the recovery process, that I stopped taking my medications. Medication is a choice for consumers and always should be, but that choice should be weighed heavily against how you think you might be able to manage without them. I made the mistake of discontinuing use of the med, as well as no longer seeing my psychiatrists, and at an early stage of recovery from a mental illness, in which medications along with therapeutic guiding could have started my journey towards recovery with a better outlook than what I would eventually endure.

Many times we as consumers are motivated into keeping engaged in our recovery by keeping ourselves healthy, doing this so that we might be able to help others with their own battles in life and recovery. In our experiences, we have gained a unique sense of empathy towards others, and in our own struggles, distraught by them, like to see others succeed. This is where I found my next motivator, where I was now, back under the care of a physician, taking my medication, and now in therapy as well. With all of these positive practices of mental health recovery at hand, I took on the responsibilities of a job coach for people with developmental disabilities, with the goal in mind of eventually becoming a caseworker for people with developmental disabilities, while at the same time being enrolled in college, now studying rehabilitation. My motivation was now to help alleviate the symptoms and keep myself active in recovery, not only to find success in life as before, but to do it with the simultaneous aspect of my chosen field being a calling. A calling where I could serve others and help in any way I could to better their lives. This I was successful at as well and it led to many opportunities for me, working and learning about everything from job development, to being a caseworker on a mental health team at a local clinic. I learned much about recovery at this point and was practicing it daily, taking it on as a responsibility.

Still, things in life happen to us which we have no control over, or are unexpected, sometimes referred to as traumatic events. This event came to me while I was working at the mental health clinic and became diagnosed with a neurological disorder. This disorder known as dystonia was greatly interfering with my work duties, and the regular treatments for the disease were working to no avail. My last option was a new treatment which involved brain surgery, which I underwent, and although helping the physical ailment I suffered with, the experience itself threw the world as I knew it into disarray. I went from stability in life and health to losing my job and the destruction of my marriage, all of which would wind me up in yet another hospital, with the end result a three month commitment at a state psychiatric facility.

It can be seen from my experiences how unexpected events happen to us as consumers, ones that we sometimes have no control over. This being a prime example, and although working on my recovery, I had not put into order the things necessary to de escalate a crisis such as this, where during such a crisis, the ones that cared and loved me did not know what else to do to help me, except by a commitment to a state hospital. This just further proves that we as consumers must continue in our recovery and as it is a life long illness so should our recovery initiatives, involving everyone in our lives with the knowledge of our disease, the ways in which we prefer to be helped, and the avenues with which to seek that help.

This being the most drastic of psychiatric events I had undergone, resulting in a combined total of six months of hospitalization, five of that consecutive, I again needed another motivator to get me out of the state I was in mentally, and the somatic effects the illness was having upon me. This time I had an unusual motivator of survival, along with wanting to make amends to others, as well as myself. This is where it was most important for me. While pleasing my loved ones by coming to terms with my limitations both physical and mental, I also had the motivator of wanting to please myself, by enjoying life and deciding to fully understand my illness, taking time for myself to process emotions and heal scars, while at the same time living in the moment and making memories.

As a consumer on the road of recovery, everyone's motivators are going to be unique to that individual. They might come naturally, or out of choice henceforth coming to being. As this chapter started out with an affirmation of sorts, so too can you start your motivation in that way. Finding the right affirmation which keeps positivity and motivation seeping out your veins and encourage yourself in the belief that it is possible. Every day is a new day with new struggles and new rewards. Remember that our first priority is taking care of ourselves, so that then we might take care of others and be helpful to those around us, as well as actively involved in the present moment, making memories with those in our lives. Remember in each step that we take in our recovery, to reflect upon the motivators we had at different times, where we can utilize them and gain from what we learned at that point in our journey. When we are first motivated to become involved in recovery, then we are in the right direction. For us as mental health consumers, it is sometimes hard to find motivation due to the prolonged injury our illness has had upon us and the want to give in is in pain. So to, here is where the importance of involving others in your motivations takes place as important. Our support systems however they may be set up, can serve us in rooting us on, giving us comfort, and at times simply taking care of our needs. Here too can be the importance of peer support, as engaging with people who have with you the common thread of a mental illness and the struggles and victories that go along with it can be a great outlet.

While facilitating groups at a mental health clinic a key topic, I found that as a unique people, being that we all suffer from a similar illness, we all have found the ability to look for some type of motivation to keep us engaged in recovery. Sometimes I found it interesting that while therapists try to beat around the bush about the subject of becoming motivated, in the hope that we come to that conclusion on our own, instead when we as consumers meet in group with the support of our peers that instinct for motivation comes naturally. I have seen success from people in the system with severe persistent mental illness, to people who utilize the private care system who have gained from the involvement in peer support activities. Whichever way we are divided into these separate groups, these same principles apply, no matter our level of functioning in society, or the stage of recovery we are currently in.

Perhaps the greatest motivator of all for us as consumers is the want to be symptom free. Once we take on the recognition that we have an illness and seek help with overcoming it, then our recovery is set into motion. Symptoms do not go away overnight, or in a few days like the common flu. It takes dedication and work on our part, as well as help from others. This being an important motivator should keep us with the mindset of continually working to overcome our illness, and reach the recovery as it is seen by us as individuals. Finding the motivation is just the start of a process that will find you in a state of growing as a person, becoming healthier and achieving desired roles, all of which are motivations for recovery. As in my different stages of finding motivators, it is important not to stop the journey there. Instead we should apply what motivates us by continuing on in our recovery journey, and following through gaining useful knowledge along the way.

Taking a look at what motivates you. Sometimes as mentioned it's helpful to write down a list of things or people or dreams in your life that keep you going. This is also a good place to find those that might be valuable to us as supporters.

Chapter Two

Outlook of Hope

When an individual is faced with a dilemma or conflict in their life which is in need of a resolution, hope is a functional aspect of the human emotion which comes into existence. We, as consumers/survivors, find that this hope manifests itself in many forms:

• wants in regards to relief of symptoms,

• acceptance of life's circumstances,

• acceptance of who we are as individuals,

• and the promise of a better outlook in relation to how we might be currently feeling anxiety over something preoccupying us at the time.

Hope is one of the foundations by which we, as consumers, engage in recovery; and for many of us, it is the starting point by which we gage our initial recovery outlook. This foundation helps us find meaning as to what we hope will transpire as we take on the responsibility of recovery.

In looking at hope, we see that it has an innate healing quality. In our journey of recovery, we can use it as a temporary remedy to the anxieties, symptoms, and situations in which we may currently find ourselves in life. We create the hope within ourselves by looking inward and being self-aware of how we want to feel, live, and grow. We focus on these things, as we hope in them and turn our fixations towards achieving them. This brings a natural relief in our minds from the frustrations and other symptoms we may have from depression, to a delusional state of being, as well as the physical symptoms which accompany mental illness. When applied in the context of escaping from our anxieties in a positive manner, it could be said that it is the greatest, natural, stress relief known to the human race.

Many of us may have come out of a hospital environment and sometimes regress. We may feel that we are left with no other option but to go back into that environment when we feel that need of care is required. While these institutions

serve their purpose in getting us to a point where we are stable enough to

maintain ourselves in our own journey of recovery outside their walls, they do not

go over and beyond; and they are years behind the community sense of

obligation and belief that recovery is indeed possible. In turn, we often find

ourselves feeling dehumanized by the treatment we receive while in their

confines. The strict down-talking type customer service we receive from the

people that are there to help us to recover from hurting emotions, the sense of

imprisonment and loss of freedom from their locked walls, and the monotonous

routine by which medication and minimal standards of nutrition and hygienic

facilities are given, leave us, upon release, with a state of confusion about what

the world thinks of us by the way we have just been treated.

Now, such is not true of all of these hospitals, but studies have shown that the

hospital system of care does indeed induce that feeling of dehumanization in

consumers and leaves us suspicious of the system as a whole. It is up to us not to

let that get us down. We must turn to hope and the avenues of community help

that are there for us. As we travel down our journey of recovery, we must find

solace in the position that the community health systems have taken. They are looking towards consumer input into care, individualized person-centered treatment, peer-support groups and activities, and the factual belief that one does recover from a mental illness.

Hope is also spiritual in its nature. No matter which way a person chooses to express that spirituality, it is a recovery principal vital to recovery. Some people meditate, some pray, others are satisfied with finding their own self-awareness. All of these are good recovery tools to use. The condition and conditioning of our spirit is something that cannot be overlooked. When our spirituality is overlooked, it leads us to having the problematic display of a down and damaged spirit, which affects our moods as well as relationships in our lives. We have the desire to feel good; and as human beings, we are a social force in nature and do not want to go down the road of isolation which brings us more pain and misery.

The way one practices spirituality is a completely personal choice. I am not saying that one should be involved in a spiritual fellowship in the form of a church, synagogue, mosque, or any other of the religious affiliations we know exist. However, studies have shown that individuals engaged in recovery who are also active with a religious, spiritual affiliation, have a greater chance at reaching their goals and maintaining their own recovery.

We should look towards applying hope in our lives. We do this by first setting those hopeful dreams and aspirations on paper or in our memory bank. Then, set goals and outline how to attain them. Hope then is put into action by our activities which bring us closer to the hopes that we had in mind for ourselves. Through this action, taking one step at a time, we then are able to gauge our progress of recovery as well as put into motion our recovery through the actions we take. Thus, we are working recovery by engaging in healthy life choices, as we move towards the whole goal, which is recovering from a mental illness.

I came across a man, a consumer, when I was employed at a mental health clinic and one of my duties at the time was to pick up consumers from the hospital and then take them back to the clinic where I would then do an intake and afterwards find placement for them at a boarding home most of the time. When I first met him I knew off the bat he was down. He remained silent except for some sighs here and there. He then broke the silence by asking me if we had time to go by a place he use to stay to get some of his things, hoping that they would still be there as he had departed from there not on such good terms. I agreed and we began the journey.

The journey started there and the hope that his material belongings would be there came to fruition. It would transpire to serve as a groundbreaking point by which a caseworker, being me in my peer provider role, took the extra time that most would not, thus establishing what he might had have had from the dehumanization that being in hospitals sometimes often brings and with which he shared his experiences, with the hope that the community care system would serve him in a better manner.

Our relationship moved from that of me being a service provider to us being co workers. During a time where I was employed and able to choose my team of which to bring about the great work we were attempting to accomplish, I remembered him looking for an employee to fill such a position. I had told him of the position a year ago when we first met at our encounter when I picked him up from the hospital. He had maintained his recovery with the hope that the position would one day bring about a career change for him, and that it did. He left a life of being a street hoodlum, then into the mental health system, and found great pride in securing his values so that they would not get in the way of his hope for a future where crime was not the mainstay of his existence. He became a certified peer support specialist and stayed with that company long after I moved on, as well as receiving his undergraduate certificate in supported employment.

For my own experience hope has inspired me and helped me in my own struggles as a consumer in many ways. The first is in symptom relief. I was having the racing thoughts going over and over in my head continually with no break, usually delusional in nature and this frustration would not stop. A caseworker then reminded me of the outlook of hope that I should have and did that by building it upon the strengths that already existed within me. She asked what is it that you want to do now that you are in progress with your recovery. That question was all changing for me, it brought back the motivations which I had once had about being successful and the value I placed in that, as well as my value of serving other people and the strengths I had with education and learning. I started to focus on that, my fixations were now of what I was going to accomplish with a positive attitude. They were not fixations about past events, traumatic scars that flashed over and over in my mind occupying time; I was now living in the present.

The hope that I had acted as a natural type of stress relief from being symptomatic in that way, although another step had to be made in taking action about those hoped for desires and goals, I was on the right track and it turned my negative into a positive.

One of the most valuable lessons I learned in acquiring an outlook of hope is when I faced my dilemma regarding my delusions about my religious beliefs. This is personal for me and how one in recovery goes about finding their own sense of spirituality is a personal decision for them to make. For me it revolved around Christianity and the Bible. I had ever-changing grandiose delusions about me being different characters in the Bible and I so wanted to go to church and participate, and feel like other Christians do. I had hoped that one day I would and then I got some advice from a therapist. She told me that I have a lot of knowledge about the Bible, more that she ever had, and that was strength to use. She said the Bible is written with a lot of things in mind but one of them is to give examples of people that the writers of the Bible wanted to show through identifying with the biblical figures that God knows that we all have different strengths and weaknesses and flaws about us. So I looked hopefully for an answer and that answer came to me, I could identify with the characters, not being them as I was in more irrational states of delusion, but could understand

and learn what they learned through their experiences about how to be stronger

in my faith. The result was that this dispelled a lot of my delusions and I was able

to go back to practicing my spirituality the way I enjoyed it. It was also helpful in

coming to this conclusion when I worked as a peer support specialist and

facilitated a group where a young man after months of group work revealed this

same trouble. I explained my outlook on it, which he grasped and began outlaying

his own unique recovery efforts in that.

Having hope that we will as consumers succeed to a stage of recovery, one that

we are comfortable in, which affords us the quality of life that we long for, is an

all important aspect in the overall scheme of recovery. We need to have hope in

ourselves that things will get better, as we see that hoping in the things that we

want bring about action. That action would be in applying it to our lives, focusing

on the dreams we have and with a motivating force driving us keep on believing

in that hope. The assistance we gain in interaction with our caseworkers and

peers as we attend groups and activities show us that there are many like us who

for some reason, etiology unknown as of yet, have had their lives altered by this

disease we generically call mental illness. We can see in these places that they all are in different stages of recovery, and that we too, being part of their journey

can aid us as well. Remember to nurture your hope by constantly reminding

yourself of your motivators behind its essence, and remember that we will never

give up hope!!

Chapter Three

Triggers

We all have things in life that somehow tend to put us into states of anxiety. They can come in the form of a person, or place, which triggers a memory, or even coincidental re-enforcers that make us believe to be true that which is not. Some things trigger in our mind thoughts of happiness and comfort. The objective to living healthily is to know the difference between the two types of triggers, and then learn how to effectively cope when a trigger arises. We as human beings cope with our emotions, which are then played out in our behavior. So learning what our triggers are, and how to process them, not avoid them, because avoidance is not always possible, is a must in our individual journey of recovery. When we grasp the effect they have upon us, then we can proceed with a spirit of adaptation to our environment, as we know that mental illness sometimes have environmental triggers.

A trigger which produces good feelings and emotionally engulfs us to the platitudes of love type emotions, which are happiness, joy and laughter, we should utilize and aspire to keep them in our lives, as they promote good mental health and cathartic experiences. When considering the triggers in our lives that induce anxious feelings and the platitudes of fear emotions, which are anger, loneliness, guilt and shame, a few among the many, we need to be aware that these are not bad emotions, but rather we should look towards them as emotions that need to be expressed in a healthy way. If they are not noted and expressed, then an unhealthy expression will take place over time, as the buildup of the emotion now is at its boiling point, and we act out the feelings caused by our emotions in a negative way.

Pinpointing your triggers, good and bad, will help you to determine the way you perceive and engage your recovery. Being aware of what they are takes a process of self evaluation, and an in-depth look at what truly drives you to feel a certain way. There are several skills which can enable you to find these triggers. An often times thought of as a simple one is the charting and journaling about who in life or what in life makes you feel a certain way, or aggravates your symptoms. Be honest and open with yourself as you write these down, and don't forget to write down the good ones down as well, as they are also vital to recovery. Remembering your experiences in life and things that relate to it, we sometimes bring back what might be seen as a negative memory, causing an anxious reaction, and although emotionally exhausting, it is a process of becoming aware that will aid you in learning how to cope with your triggers. One example is if a certain smell or song brings back an old painful memory that may cause you to become down and depressed. Another is a coincidental re- enforcer that might initiate delusional type symptoms, because something on a topic someone has said has brought into remembrance, through similarities in your own delusional thought process, that may open up your mind to that way of thinking again.

When you start to realize what these triggers are then the next step is to find ways that you can process them in a way that is beneficial to your mental health and advantageous in your recovery. If there are certain events, songs or memories that bring you happiness, joy and laughter, or people or associations that promote that wealth of healthy emotions in your life, then make a note to be centered in around those so that you might benefit from them. Also be aware that the fear emotions are not necessarily bad. Fear is most likely a poor word for the emotions of loneliness, anger, confusion or guilt, but we as a distinct people, in that we all share in similar symptoms stemming from a diagnosis of a mental illness, are not a people of fear. We have proven this as we have overcome and persevered in so many ways to have that belief. But for the purpose of labeling them, these fear based emotions are not bad emotions, rather emotions that need to be expressed, and finding and pinpointing the triggers that set off those emotions is important. If there is something that makes you angry than use skills such as communication to release that pent up energy, talk it out with someone, a peer or even a therapeutic aide. You can also exercise and reflect spiritually on how this emotion of anger was sprouted and then logically find a way to alleviate it so that it no longer has a control over the way you live life.

Remember that while emotions are based on the way we feel, they can also be dissected through logical explanation. A trauma may have occurred in your life, as we recognize that mental illnesses are traumatic events. The acceptance of that trauma, and then the commitment to shedding it off from yourself, and working towards working the triggers that inflict the memories into positive ways to express yourself, help to alleviate the pain caused by an event or person. Having a foothold of logic gives us reason for being, and reason for our expressions. It helps us, when at times we may have been living in an altered state of reality, as the social norm sees it, to regain that reality where we can function without being symptomatic and fixated on the emotional turmoil caused by these traumatic events. When we logically put into explanation our feelings and thoughts, we then have the power to put order into our lives and see things the way they are, as we are now in touch with our emotions and values. Taking this step towards reasoning and rationalization brings us closer to becoming self aware and allow us to further our recovery, when the time is right, to examine our values, which are the things we consider important in our life, and proceed with a spirit of assuredness of who we are.

Knowing our triggers and the process that it entails leads us, as consumers, to a greater sense of empowerment. This empowerment comes as we are engaged in recovery and utilizing the people and tools that are given to us, as well as the natural ones. We are empowered to make decisions in regards to controlling our feelings, and in a healthy way expressing our emotions, both the ones associated with fear, and love, as neither of them should be looked at as being negative. In our new found empowerment, we then are opened up to a world of strengths that we can now see exist in ourselves as survivors of an illness, and utilize those strengths in the areas that we desire to find accomplishment and meaning.

One of the most common mistakes we make when assessing our triggers is to focus on only identifying the negative ones. While those are important in learning the process of healing, when we forget about allowing ourselves to be aware of the positive type triggers, we rob ourselves of joy and the possibility of making good memories. Reflecting on times in our lives where in the events, or people, or things associated with them that make us feel good is vital to recovery. Sometimes we get so used to feeling down and unhealthy that we forget what it is like to feel good, or we consider it a strange and unwanted feeling when it occurs not knowing how to cope with it.

I found this in my own journey of recovery at one point. I was isolating, a common symptom among many of us, and when my loved ones would have to actually force me to go and participate in an event, of which I wanted no part, just to be left alone in my misery, I was upset and knew I would just not have a good time. Such an occasion was at the Fort Worth stock show rodeo where my dad had gotten good seats for the event. We went and even the journey to our seats was exciting, watching the cowboys practice their rides, the rodeo clowns in their getups telling jokes, but it had been a long time since I had enjoyed something, having had a dull affect for the past few years as a negative symptom of schizophrenia. These feelings I was having at that moment were strange, not because I had never had them, although the event was new to me, but because it had been such a long time since I did that I had forgotten how the body reacts towards good feelings and the acceptance of my mind in participating in enjoyment was something that I had to relearn. This I did over the course of many months, which started with that eventful night, full of excitement, which brought so much joy back to my life as before my diagnosis, as before I was a very outgoing person who enjoyed being more outside or at events then isolating shut up inside a house.

A consumer I was assigned to on my caseload when I was working as a caseworker at a mental health clinic in Dallas had long since lost his sense of enjoyment, and found that instead through the use of drugs. I took it upon myself to show him what it would be like to actually have fun, I called it social training, and asked my supervisor if I could take him to the putt putt game park to enjoy a day there and let him budget out his money, of which at the time we were the payee, so that he could manage and learn how to afford such an outing. He agreed and the consumer and I went. It was truly a real first for him, not only in the feelings that come and learning how to cope with the good sense of triggers that evoke those feelings but also with actually going to such a place. There was a smile on his face from ear to ear and it was hard to eventually get him to leave. He enjoyed this experience and said that he wanted to do it again, and I let him know that he could, but the money that he was spending on drugs he would have to save. We went a few more times before the consumer had a relapse, but I know that seed was planted there for him, that he might come back to it and remember the fun ,and the feelings of joy it brought, someday when time was right in his recovery. He might even eventually hope to reach that point again, acting as a motivator to stay clean and engaged in recovery and then his good trigger would work in a positive way for him.

Of course the other important aspect of knowing our triggers is also to be aware of the ones that cause us anxiety as well. This is important, so as not to shy away from the trigger itself, but rather to process it, so that it no longer has a control over you. Unfortunately when I was a peer specialist at a clinic running peer groups, I was a trigger for one of the consumers. At the time I did not know this was the case, and the group was disrupted by watching someone painful past and unhealed trauma unfold before their eyes. During that time it was just written up as an incident report. However, I did not want to leave it at that; showing care for the consumer in follow up is very important. So at the clinic one day when our paths crossed and I found that she was in a better state of being, she apologized to me, and I in return accepted but stated that it was good recovery to apologize, taking responsibility for your actions, but none was necessary as I am in a position of understanding as a peer and as a provider. She thanked me and I asked her what was wrong and if she would like to discuss it. She revealed that I looked, talked and most likely walked like one of her abusive ex husbands. Therefore I was a trigger in a position that was there to help her overcome her disease. We discussed it further and I assured her that I was not her ex husband, told her where I was from, and disclosed some things to her about my journey of recovery. She then opened up by letting me know that her thought for me was that she did not look at me that way, as a peer, she saw me instead as someone in authority, which in itself is a common trigger for some. We gained trust with one another and she eventually came back to the group as well as participated very actively.

One of the ways that I got this consumer back to group and the understanding of that fact that I was not her ex husband was though logic. I showed her my driver's license, with my name; I told her where I grew up, far from where she lived. Logic can help explain a lot of things and can come in handy with identifying the emotions that you have when triggers arise. We can give logic to our feelings and thoughts no matter what our diagnosis is. We had in the past looked for reasons with a mind where hope was shattered, where motivation did not exist. If we look towards logic to explain things instead of allowing our symptoms to, then we are on the right track. Sometimes even looking at our own symptoms and logically explaining why they are gives us the reason as to why we are; looking in that direction is helpful as well. Breaking down what makes us feel a certain way by where it starts or what trigger causes it, or breaking down it we are delusional by assessing the trauma which accompanies when we have those thoughts, are all ways in which we can incorporate logic. We can't always run from our triggers, especially when they have moved their ways into our minds in the process of thinking, then they are always there. So learning to cope with the bad ones, and learning to allow the good ones to give you hope will bring you closer on your journey towards recovery.

Chapter 4

Investigation of Illness

As people with a mental illness it is important that we remember that we are individuals first. It is also as equal importance that the people who serve us in rehabilitation make the effort to see us in that light as well. We may be diagnosed with an illness which bears a name, but one great quote I have heard is uplifting and those can be words to live by. In making sure that our illness does not have us, it is important to in a sense know our foe which sometimes causes so much grief. Thus it is important that we as consumers take it upon ourselves to know all there is to know about our particular illness through investigating all aspects of it. By looking into its causes or etiology, its symptoms and coping strategies, and the different treatment options available to us, it is vital to make an effort to be educated about our illness, and by doing that then we know the effects it has upon our lives.

The big word for this type of consumer involvement, and a responsibility of a rehabilitation professional, is known as psycho education. There are many different facets to psycho education, but the main premise is to make the consumer and their loved ones who are in their support network aware of all aspects regarding treatment and specified illness.

One of the things which we as consumers should be aware about and investigate is first and foremost our specific illness. We do this after being diagnosed and agreeing with that diagnosis, often times broad, through research. There are several avenues available to us, from books found in stores, pamphlets in mental health clinics, the internet and much more. In the process of this we also want to be aware of the professionalism of the information, as some can be biased and others opinionated. When we find the right one which fits into our lifestyle and is congruent with our own understanding of our illness by our own experiences, then we can use that as a guide, one which can give us answers, coping skills, and sometimes even hope and comfort.

Another important aspect of us as consumers engaging in investigation of our illness deals with knowing all there is to know about the mental health system and the services we use. Again through research, word of mouth, or even support groups where we speak with others who have been in the system longer and would gladly show us the ropes are good resources to use in identifying where to find the information which will help in determining what to expect from those who serve us.   When we know how things work then we are more equipped to make sure that all the resources available to us in regards to assisting us in reaching the goal of recovery are taken advantage of. While it is the rehabilitation professional's role to guide us, it is also of equal importance that we engage in the process ourselves, thus taking on the responsibility of recovery, a responsibility to our loved ones, society, and most importantly ourselves.

Another facet of investigating our illness comes with knowing the reasons behind it, or the etiology. There are many different philosophies and we as consumers must choose between them or incorporate portions from each one to be at ease and satisfied with our own outlook. The biological model of mental health treatment weighs heavy on the assumption through scientific tests that the root cause can be found through genetics and brain chemical makeup. The treatment then for this has arisen in the use of medications that serve to promote the different neurons in order to get them to work more efficiently for us.

There is the environmental aspect of how our surroundings and events that have taken place in our life are the root cause for onset of illness. This is whereby we realize that mental illnesses are traumatic events and the pinpointing of our symptoms are defense mechanisms to the way we cope with the emotional scars. Other facets of the environmental model are drug use, child abuse, and other unexpected or repeated events. The treatment for this is twofold, first with the use of medications and then also combined with that therapy to solve the mysteries of our symptoms, behaviors, and how they all combine to produce an illness that may have made functioning in life impaired for a moment.

One more detail of investigating your illness is involving family members. Having a strong support network is vital to recovery and if it is not your family members then friends you may have that care enough to get involved or fellow peers that you have had the opportunity to get to know and rely on one another. In any case it can involve family history of disease for possibly etiology, or history of environmental settings from friends as they, with your allowance, give a more detailed record of daily routines and past histories of events.

When we put into motion the investigation of our illness then we are fully accepting what we are faced with in life, yet have control over it. We are in touch with our traumas and are making learning ways to put them behind us, through communication skills that we have actively put into place with our caseworkers and support systems, and all of this has led up to activating our recovery.

I had a peer whom I served that had burned all of his bridges with his family members. He was a consumer who self medicated, using drugs as a means by which to control or rather curtail the symptoms at the present moment, but they would come back with a vengeance, and along with them would come the agonizing self defeat of using once again and the added definition of being an addict.

The way by which I came into his life was while I was working as a case manager at a mental health clinic with a relatively small number of consumers on my caseload. He had just been released from jail, on a drug possession charge, and I was there to take him to what would be his home. I was unfamiliar with that place but it was a halfway house which he had once been a resident of and was very uncomfortable with the placement. I attempted to find him an alternate placement immediately but to no avail; he was stuck there for the weekend at least.

When I went there that Monday, he was gone. I looked around the streets for him in spots he might be and then I got a call on my cell phone. It was him calling from a pay phone and he immediately went into the predicament he was in and how the negative peer pressure from other residents at the halfway house had sent him on a drinking binge. He felt terrible physically, mentally and spiritually. His emotions were all a wreck and he was uncertain what to do. He wanted to be clean and sober and he wanted to go along with the medical treatment plan given to him by the intake coordinator, to at least be a model client. Unfortunately that is sometimes what some people in the mental health field refer to individuals with a mental illness as looking at the disease and not the illness.

I felt his pain, I had been there before myself, and I was going to do everything that I could possibly do to help him in his circumstances. The first thing that I did was to get him into an addiction center where he spent a week. This time allowed him to think about his goals for recovery and me some time to regroup and see how I might go about helping him find better supports.

These better supports came to me in the fact that he wanted to get back in touch with his parents, who had long since lost track of him and counted the loss of the son to the streets. This really hit home for me, and when he called I identified myself as a case worker and asked if it was at all possible that we meet and talk about their son's future. They agreed, which both the consumer I was helping and I were delighted by. What the eventual outcome was after an afternoon of psycho education which I gave to the parents, was a better understanding of the mental health system, a better understanding of their sons' illness, his disease of addiction and hope for them that he could gain a foothold on all of them. This hope came in the form of, after all the information had been given to them, I shared my own experiences with recovery, which were very similar, and them seeing me in a position which helped others gave new light to the situation that had been dealt with for many years.

The consumer also being enlightened by his disease found a place called the Oxford House where his parents agreed to pay for the housing. It was an addiction house where members learned to live drug free together. They were on the right track. With his ambition and one of his basic needs met he wanted to know more about his disease of bi polar and the etiology of where it all came from. He attended counseling sessions at the clinic, group workshops, and through the outcome of this all he decided to attend training for peer support. Although he did not proceed with finding a placement as a peer specialist, he did gain a lot of useful information which could be used to maintain his recovery for years to come. He found through his own ambition and investigation of his illness the motivation to stay in recovery. He put forth his recovery into motion further by applying for and finding a position as a line cook at a local restaurant.

Chapter 5

Objectives and Goals

We as consumers, when we get to a place of finding our motivation, learning what our triggers are and ways to process them, should then look with an outlook of hope towards establishing roles in life that we wish to participate in or the reestablishment of those that have been damaged or lost. More than that though, we look at our recovery now as a turning point by which to achieve and maintain a healthy lifestyle, and a quality of life which we are content with. In doing this it is vital that we begin to reestablish the way we look at bringing about our accomplishments. We have established our hopes and aspirations and now we need to be engaged by making steps in fulfilling them. Along with these hopes and aspirations, should also come into play our desire to achieve recovery from a mental illness. With these put together in their entirety we come to find that it is a non linear approach to recovery that we are looking towards, where recovery for us is based on individual needs for a variety of life's circumstances, as well as our goal of recovery.

This for many of us starts at the intake portion when we have by for whatever reason forced, or by our own will found the motivation to seek assistance in our journey of recovery. It is important that we make note that this is our journey and although many times assisted by those of out therapeutic team, it is vital to make our input known and confirmed by them as how we would like to proceed. This journey at first begins with small steps sometimes, writing down and working on achieving smaller goals, with still the big picture in mind, but with a measurable outcome so that we can see change happening in our lives and that change and progress can produce feelings of accomplishment. It is important also for us as consumers to remember to allow time for healing. This may mean several different things, from getting assistance in the roles that you do have in life from those in your support system, to taking time off of work and using the ADA guidelines to help us with that. Now these are just suggestions but the point is that healing sometimes finds itself being in the background to the other things that we do in life, and if we don't take that time to heal then the progression of our disease will continue in the same areas or others.

In setting goals it is important to remember that they go hand in hand with objectives. Your objectives are activities which you do in order to reach your goals. For many of us the first goals that we often find ourselves in need of are the very things that are necessary for everyday living. Things like shelter, resources for food, and the things vital to sustaining life. These of course are the first things that should be considered and a caseworker is a great resource for that. We can also learn to lean on our natural resources if we belong to a church who helps those with food or living situations, and other resources outside of the mental health system, keeping in mind that one of the overall goals of recovery is to achieve stability outside the use of the mental health system and lean on the community in our interactions with society towards achievement of our satisfied quality of life we desire.

Once our essential needs are met, if they are not already, then the next step can be to focus on symptom relief, which is the case for many of us and a big motivator towards the need to be engaged in recovery as well. The goal then is evident: alleviation of symptoms; the objectives then are the things we do in order to make that a reality. Medication and the management of them are often times our first source. So our time spent with the doctor should be productive by us taking the effort to taking the time to write down in an effective manner the information that we know the doctor would like to know which is what he makes his decisions based on. These things range from symptoms, and us having the ability to know when and judge the severity of them, as well as times that they most frequently occur. Letting the doctor know of any major changes in our lives that could be environmental reasons of being symptomatic; also important is letting the doctor know in all honesty your intake of caffeine, nicotine and even drugs as all of these can play factors in mood and thought symptoms. In doing this the doctor can make better judgments of how we can be treated. Also all of these things are talked about during clinical meeting between your caseworker and the doctor treating you with them working in tandem for the betterment of your outcome.

We should make ourselves informed about the different coping techniques and practices that are available for us to use to fight the onslaught of symptoms. A good resource for this can be your caseworker in teaching you skills training in that area and by doing your own research most days on the internet and learning about your particular diagnosis and what others have used or other proven methods that you can try and see if they work for you. All of this is what is called being engaged in recovery and taking these steps then leads to new experiences with new strengths by which to progress on the road to recovery.

There are other goals that you may wish to implement in your recovery at this stage and by making sure to outline the objectives for you to reach those means you are keeping your recovery in motion. Remember that although you start off small you still have the need and want to look forward with the hopes that you have and how you would like your life to be lived in a healthy way, and by the decisions you have made in which way you want your path to go. This is the overall goal setting. With most of us, one of the overall goals will likely be recovery from our illness and the symptoms that aggravate us, but along with that are the goals by which we see ourselves participating in life, our roles, our pastimes, and our spiritual growth. In looking at the overall goal, the big picture of these things, make your objectives step by step with measurable realistic amounts of time for you to achieve them. The end result will be that your dedication to your engagement in recovery will bring forth the fruitfulness in your life that you have hoped for as well as worked for.

Many times we as consumers get stuck in this portion of recovery. It is by no fault of our own, we have all the good intentions, wanting to progress in our recovery, and achieve the things we desire.   But where we can get lost is in paying attention to the big picture, how nice it all looks, seems and hopes to be, and we forget about the tedious steps that we must take and the reliance of the completion of them in order to live in that big picture or goal.

This is a part of recovery that is vital to being involved in life's moments and where growth occurs. By taking on these new responsibilities that push us farther towards that goal, we are thus becoming that person who that goal is intended for. By living in the manner that makes that goal possible and by paying attention to the detail that when it is achieved we find the feelings of thankfulness, and accomplishment which the process has led us to become.

I found myself stuck in this phase for a time in my own recovery. I would sit and do nothing but daydream about what I wanted to accomplish. While this did help me get off the topic of other symptoms that were held down by this part of my journey, I was still going to bed at night and waking up the same person, with nothing achieved and nothing gone forward towards that achievement. A simple yet often times shrugged off tool which I used, was journaling. I wrote down all the things I wanted to achieve or what I wanted to become in life now that my symptoms were under control and I had an outlook of hope about recovering from my illness and doing the things that I desired in life, instead of dwelling upon the sickness itself.

This journaling led to setting objectives down on paper of what I needed to do on a daily or weekly basis to achieve what I wanted to achieve. I then being old fashion bought a daily planner and started to put down everything that came to mind that I needed or wanted to do filling up the entire daily and weekly space. It wasn't overwhelming, having that much on there to accomplish, due to the fact that I knew myself that these were just objectives and that if I accomplished one or more I was gaining ground. The ones I did not accomplish would then be written down for the next days' activities.

Following this path I found that I was starting to become active in my recovery; not only was my recovery in motion, I was playing a more vital role and living life as I did recovery, making memories as I went along with the things I did and the people I came across, and boosting my self esteem as I saw myself engaged in not only my recovery but in life in general. What this led to for me was the creation of my web page where I wrote articles about mental health topics and the final draft of my first book Downward Spiral Uphill Battle.

Chapter 6

Neglecting Our Needs

Due to the debilitating effects of the generalized disease of mental illness, we sometimes succumb to neglecting our own needs as we are faced with the onslaught of symptoms accompanying the disease. We find ourselves exhausted not only by the somatic effects of the disease itself, but also mentally and physically from battling the symptoms on a daily basis, Therefore it is not uncommon that we wind up showing ourselves neglect in areas that if they were attended to would be beneficial for our overall health, mental as well as physical. One of the main things consumers often have in common in neglecting ourselves in our health is hygiene. It is amazing how we go for years on end starting at an early age, brushing our teeth and showering and using lotion to take care of our skin, and then once we are hit with the illness this all goes out the window. Poor hygiene is in fact very common among mental health consumers, and is at some point something that needs to be addressed. It springs from the negative symptoms of lack of care, lack of energy, and again plain exhaustion from the mental illness. It seems so simple and sometimes our loved ones just do not understand it. However at this point our recovery is in motion and the next step of activating that recovery can start here. Engaging actively in a daily routine and making sure that your ADL's (activities of daily living) are being met.

Where do we start if our activities of daily living and the function of such things are so distraught? The answer can be simple; we make it a priority, and find motivation for us to partake in them. With hygiene, once we engage ourselves in that task we will soon find right out of the gate how much better we feel from our efforts at being clean. Another motivator besides feeling good is that we want to show others around us that we care enough about ourselves, and them seeing that shows them that we care also enough to succeed in the responsibility of recovery. Sometimes this leads to praise towards our actions and the involvement of the consumer and the support system members working in tandem to make the quality of life for each involved better.

Another skill associated with ADL'S is making preparations throughout the day to ensure your nutrition needs are met. Perhaps the biggest motivator of all for this is hunger. We in this society have come to promote eating as pleasurable, not necessarily for nutrition purposes, and if we start with the pleasure then the nutrition is a goal that can be worked on later. The fact that we at points in our recovery, especially starting out, do things like skip meals because of not wanting to prepare them, or forgo a meal because we would rather have our nicotine and rely on that and coffee to sustain us. All these are habits we must break; not only is nicotine and coffee a terrible source of a notorious meal, it makes your moods fluctuate through their drug induced states on the chemical makeup of our brains. Another motivator for moving on to nutritious food preparation can be that you want to get into that swimsuit for the summer, or that you might be able to come off expensive medicine for diabetes.

Taking care of our living environment is essential as well. The reasons for lack of ADL's has been noted, but now that our recovery is in motion, we are moving towards the activation stage, which is going to require more awareness by us as consumers, the ability to apply skills taught and natural ones to us. It is not uncommon for someone not to want to clean or do household chores; nobody enjoys it regardless of mental well being or not. But, partaking in this activity will one be positive as we find that the expenditure of energy leaves us with a good feeling of accomplishment and our bodies with a good feeling of being active for a period of time, and two we will see a change in who we are as individuals as we put back together through order the things that had become disorganized in our lives. We can look back now and reflect on our growth thus far, and give ourselves our own praise, which will hopefully keep us motivated and nurture our hope by seeing that through putting things into motion and now on the verge of becoming more active in our recovery, the dreams and aspirations that we have will come into being and the feelings of accomplishment will surface as well, just as they have done here.

ACTIVATE

In this second phase of recovery we are starting to become more active in our recovery. Being engaged in recovery takes action on our part and knowing which areas to focus on is of importance, as it keeps us centered. Anything undertaken is done so through action, so too is recovery as it is sought out by us.

During this phase we learn to apply concepts such as acceptance and focus on the proper ways which will benefit us as we learn to communicate our concerns to others as well as communicate to others our feelings and emotions, the importance of processing those emotions and relation they have and mental illness has towards trauma. The concept of healing mental illness as opposed to maintaining its symptoms is examined.

The importance of self awareness is examined and tools by which to make that come to fruition are given. The concept of knowing what our values are, and the importance of living by those values so that we are not at war within ourselves by living against that which we consider important, taking the time to manage these activities and our mental illness as a whole is examined. As we activate our recovery we are gaining ground towards the goal of recovery as how we visualize it to be and take place in our life.

Chapter 7

ACCEPTANCE

Having the ability to be content in life is a character trait that promotes healthy

living. Learning to be content helps us accept life's circumstances. Contentment

works to alleviate stress, and this is beneficial for almost everyone regardless of

one's role in life. Acceptance is a big part of learning to be content. It can be

looked at from several different angles in life. When unscheduled, unplanned or

unexpected circumstances occur, we need to be flexible and accepting of these

events or circumstances simply because there is no other choice. Our reaction

can lead us to handle properly and successfully these circumstances or promote

negative reactions such as anger, unrest and confusion. While we may not be able

to control the circumstances, we can control our reactions to these

circumstances. From minor inconvenience to major trauma we experience these

difficulties and surprises in life and they affect us physically, socially or mentally.

We need not only to assess these changes in our life experiences but also the changes in our character and personality. To be in control of these changes, we need to learn to accept our circumstances and the pressures of acceptance that is placed in our lives. By accepting our difficulties, accepting our challenges and accepting our realities this allows us to not be detoured in the search to place blame, or feel sorry for ourselves or waste precious moments trying to escape the abyss. Let us look for ways to take it for what it is; that it is a fact and reality in our lives, and find healthy ways to process whatever the content may be.

Looking at acceptance, we see that it often times leads us to escape the frustration within ourselves. We act out our denial about the content requiring acceptance. Confusion results in the processing and assessing of the problems and prevents us from being able to move forward in life because of these circumstances. At its roots is in the natural human behavior of not wanting to release control of one's own self. We try as hard as we can to hold onto that control. We end up damaging ourselves emotionally and sometimes physically, by not accepting the limitations or the realizations of the very circumstances we find ourselves in. When we give up that need for control, however, we are then given even more power and control over our lives as we gain awareness and ability to determine how we will accept and process the circumstances in which we find ourselves. Failure to properly use acceptance principles can result in setting forth lies that come with denial. We end up avoiding or shunning our experience with an event we have not yet accepted. This builds resentment not only of others but also of ourselves. What happens when we leave those feelings and the actions that we take when not having a spirit of acceptance, is a process of having control over how we perceive our situation, event or even ourselves. We are freed to grow in our own understanding of how it affects us, and allows it to become part of who we are. Instead of resentment, we find courage to change through learning and allowing our experience to guide us in the further decisions that we make.

By applying acceptance in our lives, we create a new outlook to help us grow as individuals. Some may think that acceptance is a negative word that forces us to accept life as learning to live with life as the cards that have been dealt us. Instead, we learn that acceptance is actually a word that is active and alerts us to produce change. When we apply it to the process of healing we learn that in accepting we are actually programming ourselves to a sense of understanding in relation to how the event or content is affecting our lives. When we begin to understand how it is affecting us, then we can plan and put forth the effort required and to alter the control that it has had in our lives. We start to see how our actions have led us to this event we need to accept, or how our viewpoint in life about the event or circumstances has caused us to stall in emotional growth. The next step is to learn from whatever has kept us blinded through the powers of frustration and proceed with due diligence in what we now know, how we are now new in disintegrating the denial, and how we will now proceed with a heart of understanding and the power to create change.

Acceptance is also about learning to be content in the situations life has in store for us. Through acceptance we learn how to adjust to the change that may be needed to overcome adversity. When we are content then we are not giving away control again, rather we are applying control in our lives. This allows us to not only gain acceptance of our situation, but also slowly take the morsels of hope that will keep us strong during our journey of recovery. We will know that what is now is not forever. We gain confidence and assurance as more opportunities and challenges are sent our way. Therefore, being content serves as a challenge for us to achieve awareness and alertness. This brings us to a state of your calmness in our souls, peace in our minds, and order in our lives. We are allowed to look for the opportunities that are available throughout the recovery process. We will find empowerment as we make decisions. We will experience

goals and aspirations becoming more attainable. Our roles will become more

definable and easier to fulfill as we experience acceptance.

For many years, with no treatment at times, and then with little attention paid to

my treatment as a person, not as a diagnosis, I proceeded in living my life without

the acceptance of some the behavior I exhibited and the actions that I did. I did

this by always pointing the finger, and placing blame. What this led to was a

strange delusional thought process that gave reason to the absurd behavior that I

exhibited. Instead of me being having a spirit of acceptance with being at fault

with the things I had done, I often tended to blame God, misconstrued by the

scripture that says everything is done for a reason. So I felt that everything I did

was for a reason to God, and hide the fact that I had shame or guilt from hurting

myself and the ones I loved as well as innocent bystanders along the way. It

wasn't until I accepted and with the old NA AA additive of making amends to

those who I found fault with, and then allowing acceptance about these things,

did I then gain control of the haunting thoughts. When I did I was conscious, and

proceeded to set forth to regain in my life a recovery where I accepted my mental

illness as being my concern, not others. Although there are those who live and care about us who help, I realized that it was my responsibility, and one I had to choose to take on for the rest of my life.

In a peer support group that I facilitated strictly for peers with probation or parole issues, a consumer came to terms with this process of acceptance which he had dealt with for many years. Angry at the system and not even able to go inside a public restaurant to get a hamburger, having to wear a monitor to tell the police where he was at all times, he was frustrated with the lack of freedom he had. When I engaged him with the fundamentals of acceptance he revealed that he had applied several times before to be moved off the position of being on a monitor and each time was denied. We delved deeper into this occurrence and found that he had been denied many times because he kept on missing scheduled appointments or wasn't adhering to his parole. He, through insight, came to the conclusion that he was in fact not gaining control through acceptance but rather allowing others to control him for not allowing the spirit of acceptance to sink in. He was sabotaging his own freedom because of his anger for the system and not accepting his role and the responsibilities that came with it of abiding by the rules. Throughout my tenure with the group, he had finally got off the monitor and was allowed to go eat his hamburger at a restaurant. All because he did the things required at the time and accepted that he had to do them in order to gain control in his life.

We must also be open to change and not fight with resistance things that come along with that change. We must be flexible as consumers, not letting change of circumstances deviate us from our recovery. It is a law of physics if you will, if one thing goes away put another in its place. I saw this transpire with a consumer who was under my care as I was a caseworker, and she was dealing with at that time her daughter wanting to live a life of her own and in that desire, the consumer was in need of finding a new place to live as her daughter's new life and marriage began. She was reluctant at first, not wanting the life as she knew it to change. Instead of rolling with the resistance and into a new comfort zone, she did not apply acceptance and each time a new door opened for her she was not alert and ready take advantage of the opportunity. She had several offers of other consumers willing to take on a room mate, and where it eventually led her was a boarding home where she finally was thrown out trying to manage on her own, angry and using drugs in response to the change. With the rehabilitation door open to her once again and the efforts made by many at the clinic including myself she finally was willing to accept that change along with the emotions which came along with it. With a new place in plan about how she would be in her daughter's life from now, and a boarding home where several rehabilitative services were offered, her spirit of acceptance and being flexible to change finally came through and she found success in that and went forward with her own personally journey of recovery.

Chapter 8

Communication

Communication is a key to everything that we do in life. It helps us in socializing with others, processing our thoughts and feelings, and is necessary for everyday living in how we get our needs met. Without communication we would not be able to express ourselves, and within recovery, expression of how we feel and what needs we need to be met is essential when progressing in recovery. In knowing this then it is helpful to find what might be in our way as far as communicating to others, especially in regards to our therapeutic teams who assist in that reality of recovery which we have hoped for, and accept it as our responsibility.

Our time with therapists sometimes seems very valuable as it is often seen as not as lengthy a time for us. So being able to communicate effectively during that time we have with them is important, as we see them rarely and for short periods of time. The things we need to get across to them are vital as they are concerning our feeling emotions and symptomatic troubles for which we want to find relief. So going prepared is important, and there are tools in which to make that preparation. One good tool is a log book of the time you have spent in between seeing them and up to the point where you are ready to see them again. Writing down any feelings and symptoms and rating them as to how they are affecting you will give you a source to rely on and bring about remembrance during your time with your caseworkers, peer guides, doctors, etc.

Also communication can take many forms for a consumer. One of those ways by which it manifests itself is in the form of advocating for yourself. You do this with the assurance that your voice will be heard and your needs looked at and met. With a calm assertiveness in your disposition while communicating you will gain a sense of empowerment as you see that instead of sitting back and allowing things to occur in regards to your health, you are taking action and working them towards your favor.

Listening is also a part of communication. When we are attentive listeners when others are involved with us in the process of communication, we show that we are open to suggestion and with a spirit not of closed mindedness, others will gravitate towards your willingness to be a team player in your recovery. Knowing how to listen in life also allows us to be invested in the process of learning. With learning comes more responsibilities in life as we are then equipped with the knowledge of how to make things a reality through the powers of organization and application. This then opens us up to ascertaining the responsibilities which we now have in life and gives us a sense of joy as we recognize that we are building bridges in life, maintaining them, and builds our self esteem as we move forward in life.

Communication with ones' self is an important part of growth as well. We do this by the awareness of ourselves as individuals and what is important to our spiritual growth in whatever form that may be. We practice this form of spirituality through meditation in communing with ones inner being, in which we come to realizations through its relaxation techniques that which are important to us, coming close with our feeling and emotions and how we want to communicate them in a healthy way, so that they do not build up inside of us where over time we are forced to act them out in a negative way. We practice our spirituality by finding the way we want to be perceived as to who we are in our lives and interactions with others. If we desire to have integrity then we make an effort to be strong in our beliefs and not be dissuaded by others' negative actions. If we desire to be compassionate then we show that through helping others, volunteering, and small but all important acts of kindness towards others. There are many ways in which we can communicate our spiritual nature and these are just a few.

Communication is also a two way street. We communicate with others and it is reciprocal in nature. We listen to what others deduce from our communicating and reflect that accuracy is made and that another's opinion is taken into account through understanding. We see these as consumers so vital in regards to our support systems. Support systems comprise those people or organizations that we have in our life who support us in our journey of recovery. They include parents, siblings, caseworkers, social networks, friends and others. As we communicate with them, we should do so with a spirit of regard to an appreciation of their involvement. WE notice that this disease not only affects us but the ones who are in our lives as well. With the realization that they have feelings and emotions not only in their own make up as human beings but also in regards to their position in our lives as a supporter of a person with a mental illness. When we communicate effectively with them, then we are working together, and being in a united front is more successful than not being in one. Show them compassion as we hope that they will show it for us.

As we have not only put our recovery in motion, but also activated it, we find that communication is clearly important in our roles as consumers active in our recovery. I found this to be very helpful in regards to maintaining my relationships with those in my support system. When I isolated and suffered in my disease one of two things would happen. One, they would see me suffer and I would deteriorate into my own world of thoughts, or two, I would allow everything inside me to build up and eventually explode in fits of anger, not often, but the truth is that it did happen a time or two. When I applied communication to my recovery, then and only then did my relationships begin to establish themselves and the support that I was so in desperate need of was not only there, it was offered with kindness and empathy.

Applying communication in my own illness also opened up the door to education within my support network about my disease. They started to listen no matter how off the wall the thought might have been and tried to understand or at least show support. This grew not only in receiving support but also in the areas of them establishing me as a son, a sibling, and friend. I did have an illness that I had to be consistent with in regards to recovery oriented tasks, but they were able to look past that in the sense that I was still a person in their life who they knew before illness struck and saw pass the sometimes ugly behavior that I would exhibit, or the sometimes thought of as lack of care that I gave towards achievement in life.

While I was working in my position as a peer support specialist, I was facilitating a group at one of the clinics and the topic came up about why the doctors gave us only fifteen minutes of time for our visit with them, and in that time submit us to a diagnosis. Now while I agree this time is not always sufficient and more should be done in the way psychiatrists treat us as consumers, they are physicians, who live by the rule that medication is the answer and they are treating symptoms, not a person's psyche as a whole.

In knowing that I also was able to give the peer I was working with in group some insight, which I did not know either until my time as a caseworker. That insight led him to the conclusion about how important communication is when you are in treatment time with caseworkers and others that guide you along the path of recovery. Being the way the system is now, and change is coming, but until that change is in full effect we must learn to use what we have in order to better our lives for the moment in time that we are in. In doing this all that we communicate to our therapeutic team members, once a week in most cases, is discussed with the doctor in a group setting. Treatment goals and outcomes are discussed on a per client basis, as well as many other topics. The doctor also has at his or her hand the ability to read case notes that have been taken by our therapeutic team members that guide us, whose observation and our vital input into our own recovery is observed and intervened by the specific person in charge of that intervention and planning outcome.

This information not many consumers know, as it is a behind the scenes look, as was the case with me before being behind those doors, and with my peer who was concerned before I gave him the knowledge about such happenings. This peer left more confident that things were being done on his behalf and that more time was given to him than the meager fifteen minutes that he was seen by his treating physician.

So as we with a spirit of acceptance are content with the time afforded to us by the workers in the system, make sure on our own behalf that we be avid advocates of ourselves and our needs by way of communicating all that is needed in the determinate of our care, so that we play a part in that care as we are the best historians of our disease and where it has taken us.

Chapter 9

Trauma

We know that mental illnesses are traumatic events, so it is helpful to define what traumatic events are. Traumatic events can be in the form of painful memories of tragic circumstances, loss of a person or relationship, loss of a role in life such as a job, and the inability to process poor behavior in the past. What leads us often to the development of symptoms is our unwillingness to examine our traumas and accept them as part of who we are, then the commitment, being mindful of who we are as individuals, allowing ourselves to live in the moment instead of the painful past.

Traumas often times fester and our reliance upon them is due to an attitude of refusing to allow ourselves to heal by facing what the trauma is that causes us to be symptomatic. We tend to get stuck in the past and our thoughts instead of being focused in the present, are turned towards the agonizing events that have somewhat stalled our lives' progression. Once we know what that trauma is in the process of uncovering it we can allow for healing to take place through acceptance.

—

This is based on the concept of ACT Therapy where mindfulness strategies are used in order to begin a process of health awareness and in doing so put into place the things we value in life, then move towards making sure that our behavior reflects who we are. If we are at war with ourselves and do things that are against our nature, then we are prone to get stuck in further escalating our symptoms of mental illness because we are not being consistent with ourselves.

The first step in acceptance is through practice to alleviate the reliance that our mind has on unwanted events or memories and even feelings. We as consumers do this by being aware of the event instead of holding it in. This may seem scary as these events sometimes are and the mind in mental illness works by, instead of defusing the control they have on us, keeping us trapped in that pain. This plays out in our thoughts, feelings, memories, and behavior. If a loss of a role in life for example is the source of the trauma, it can plague us in different forms. In our memories we can focus on the past and become entangled with how great our job was, how much we miss it, and how the devastation of losing it has ruined our lives. It can also cause us to bring on another symptom. It might be that we cognitively distort it, with the unwillingness to accept it and move forward and try to rationalize it as someone is out to get us or that it was some type of divine intervention causing symptoms of delusional concepts.

A big part of remaining in our illness is that we remain in our past. We as consumers can find ourselves fixated on all that had happened to us, or the people who have gone their separate ways along the way. We stay stuck in time and as such we do not participate actively in all life has to offer in the present moment. As we are now activating our recovery it is important that we understand as consumers what this means. It means that we become aware of all that is around us in the present moment, in our thoughts, our feelings, and our senses. When we do this we are able to let life's progression move us forward, and experience new feelings and events which create new memories with the aim of them being healthy and healing in nature.

I enjoy writing stories of my peers for several reasons. One of those is because I hope it will show through their own resilience that others who read about them will be inspired and have the hope and the courage that goes along with that hope to believe in themselves that they can succeed in such things too. Another reason I use examples of peers is that some people in the mental health system still believe that recovery is not possible. This means a non linear form of treatment, where measurements of recovery are based on not only the subsiding of symptoms but also the emotional health of the individual in overcoming trauma.

I had a peer who many thought of in the clinic where I worked as what they would call sometimes simply put, a problem client. I saw an amazing transformation in this person from the time I was introduced and hopefully through the present time as I am now no longer employed there. She was your prototypical stereotype of a person with mental illness. She did not care to much in the way she was dressed or how she presented in public, and she mumbled about fixations many of the times in our meetings. In fact our first meeting together in group she had a trigger about me in particular reminding her of her past husband, whom I would later find was abusive and the cause for many of her emotional scars.

That first meeting with her she ran out of the meeting room and into the lobby. I allowed her to calm down and then approached her. I told her that if I was the reason, which she made clear that it was, that she would not participate in group, I would excuse myself to not be a downfall in her own recovery. She eventually saw that I was a non aggressive person and although my looks may have reminded her of her ex husband, she was able to gather her self and apologize to me, which was not necessary at all, and return to the group.

I then by chance had a group topic which led to me and her connecting on a level that peers have the ability to do through their similar experiences and from that point on the trust bond was formed and recovery began to take place. She began to open up more, not fixate on the past, and show up looking very nice at times even in dresses, with makeup and the whole works that women sometimes like to do by means of expression. Before our time together she would not even open up to the discussion of traumas, was fearful of them, but since has allowed the healing to occur by processing them. It was difficult at times, with tears and breakdowns caused by emotions, but the cathartic experiences and the safety felt inside the trusting walls of a peer support group gave her the courage and the assistance from other peers to remain strong and work through them.

Chapter 10

Involvement in Activities

In our role as mental health consumers, we often times find ourselves out of touch with being involved in activities. Activities promote a healthy state of being, where communication skills are enhanced through participation, and a sense of belonging is found when participating with others. Activities also do not have to be with others in a social engagement and it is often a place where we as consumers find ourselves starting to implement activities, where we engage in the ones that are of interest to us that might be done alone.

If it is here that we start, we are engaging in recovery, changing our daily routine which to some of us is found typically to be curled up in a bed with the lights out in deep sadness, isolating and further instigating the feelings of loneliness. For others it could be that we isolate as well but in a manic state of psychosis, running our minds ragged with the exploits of ideas that we think we must initiate in order to make the voices in our head happy. Whatever the reason, if we turn our fixations on becoming active then we have less and less time for the symptoms to frustrate us.

Activities starting out by oneself that can be helpful are reading and getting lost in a world of imagination other than the one that plagues our minds. We can listen to music that brings us comfort and is known to be helpful in soothing the voices. Some of us like to be active with the amount of energy that we have inside of us which needs a release, and we can find that in walking or other types of exercise. Still others enjoy being creative and projects within art such as cooking or painting bring about relief of symptoms. Another way by which we can be active is to journal our thoughts, allowing everything to release out of our minds onto paper so they we can take a better look at ourselves.

We often times need a boost to start these activities, getting in touch with what our interests were before losing our function in life to a mental illness. We look towards our caseworkers at the clinics we utilize and the other members of the therapeutic teams that are suppose to provide facilitation for change and engagement in recovery. However, it is also something that we must take into our own hands. There are some ways that we can do this. One way is to remember what we learned about motivation. We all have reasons in life to be participants in activities, and when we look inwardly at ourselves and see change as helpful to others that can sometimes be a motivator. We, like all other individuals, enjoy praise for our actions. If we start our focus there in doing it for someone else then it can evolve into having the motivations for recovery into engaging in it for yourself, thus taking care of yourself, and you then have an impact on those who began to motivate you.

Once the activities have begun, then you put yourself in the position to keep things in motion by moving forward and advancing to engaging socially. The healing that has happened on your own has most likely built confidence in yourself, self awareness, and healthy energy and ideas that you might want to share with others. A simple way of becoming engaged in social roles if isolation was your previous solution is by becoming yet again a consumer in your neighborhood. By this I mean going to different stores and establishments on a routine basis. After a while you will find that the employees of those store and even some patrons that visit as regularly as you will start to strike up small conversations. Starting at first with hey how have you been, to over time giving each other glimpses into each others' life, your strengths in the communication about all the activities you are involved in which you had been participating in on your own, to simple things about how the weather is. These might not turn into long lasting friendships but what has happened now is that you have grown in your recovery and now are more confident in your ability to hold down a conversation and give input back to those who interact with you.

Once that has been achieved and if you haven't done so already, then you can take the step of becoming involved in activities within organizations that are there for the advocacy and support of consumers. These are designed to give support in group sessions, and there as a way to make friends who can also serve as a peer support system where you grow with one another under the umbrella of what you have in common, which happens to be being a consumer. Groups such as NA, AA, NAMI, and DBSA, are all rooted with fundamentals geared towards recovery, as well as an outlet for support and understanding for what each and everyone attending go through in their journey of recovery.

Another viable option towards starting to regain a foothold back in society is to do volunteer work. Many places are thankful for the time that you are able to give, and do not get upset if you need to take some time away; the position will still be there most likely when you return. The associations that you make at a place volunteering can lead into friendships where you can test your ability to incorporate a relationship into your life, and take on others' cares and needs as they take on yours. Plus there is the self esteem that volunteering builds when you are there giving of your time to help others; it is good for the human spirit and for society. In the meantime if you are not working then this experience as a volunteer looks great on a resume when the time comes for you to start looking for employment.

Another activity which should not be taken lightly is the decision to become involved romantically with someone. While many of us as consumers feel that natural need for such a relationship there are some things to consider, and questions that we as consumers ask ourselves about when is the right time. Often times we tend to think that becoming involved with someone will end all of our woes, but remember we take on other people's woes, as well as their good traits, and that should be considered first before advancing in that direction. Are you capable of taking on the worries and concerns that an intimate relationship brings in your current state of recovery? This is a question you should ask yourself. Remember that not only is your own health at risk of deteriorating but now you have involved another person's feelings as well. This is not suggested as "beware, a relationship will make you sick", because it could turn out to be a healthy one. However, we as consumers need to be aware the state our own mental health and emotions are in before we decide to merge them with someone else's.

So what can we do if we decide the time is right and we would like to pursue such a relationship of romantic involvement? First, after it has been determined that you feel you are ready, then take small steps. We all have the fear of "the other person is not going to understand my illness" or, " when is the right time to tell a person I have an illness?" as these are tough questions, and even more so with the stigma that revolves around it. So moving into the process slowly is always the best bet. Consider being friends first, then move into dating and seeing each other occasionally. The fact of your illness and when you decide to disclose it is entirely up to you; many have tried to answer when the right time is to disclose, but there truly are not firm answers. You want to be honest with the person, and hiding the truth is never good. However it is a good idea to allow someone to get to know who you are as a person, not as how society has labeled you, and you do this through the process of becoming friends, leading to dating and then on from there, where eventually disclosure is a must. Don't be worried however; often times you will find that everyone carries what they call baggage and acceptance is always a must amongst individuals who decide to carry on that type of relationship.

Although we are consumers, we are people first. People whose situation requires these things to be looked into. We sometimes need a helpful hand to lead us through this maze of hurt emotions, scared traumatic thoughts, and feelings of hurt. As we do remember that involvement in life and life's activities are meant to be enjoyed, they can seem like a large mountain to climb to regain a foothold after a traumatic event of a mental illness, but if we educate ourselves, look towards others in trusting their guidance with an outlook of hope, keep ourselves aware of our triggers and process them healthfully, then our recovery is in motion, and we know that we have the strength to prevail.

A question one consumer asked of me in a group setting was, how do we decide to date with a person who has a disability like ours, or someone who does not have a mental illness? This is a very good question and one where the answer lies in determining what your wants and needs are out of a relationship, and whether or not that person would be able to fulfill them and you reciprocate as well. I replied to her that when being with someone it is always good to make sure that your values line up with one another's, that you are a fit in that area so that you will not clash among decisions and directions in life. Also you have to ask yourself in regards to being romantically involved with another person who has a mental illness as well as yourself, you have to realize that you will be put into the position of being a support for them, and the question must be asked whether or not you can handle that type of involvement, if it will injure your own recovery or not. The answer is there is no answer. There are a set of guidelines and warnings to go by, but again relationships are another personal choice. However it is a big role in life that you will take on if you choose to do so and making sure that you are ready for that role is essential in it succeeding.

The building which housed my office while working as a peer specialist and facilitating groups was located at a community center run by the mental health agency I was working for. There are so many advantages to a person being involved in activities if a place like this is available in your area. There are several opportunities to meet people who like you have had their struggles and give support to one another. There are also activities and groups, ranging from art classes to gardening, at least at the specific one I was involved with. But more than that many of them set up a system of involvement through volunteering and allowing for roles of responsibility to be placed on consumers who are actively seeking such an opportunity. We had at our community center people who ran the snack bar, did cleaning around the center, ran the front desk and much more, which eventually turned into a paid stipend for them receiving money for the work that they had done.

There are several ways to get involved in activities and the eventual goal is to rely on the natural supports outside the realm of the mental health network, here in the community where you are involved in activities and organizations that are in line with your past times, spirituality or memberships of unique quality that you fit into. One of the goals of recovery for us is to systematically set in place all these natural supports so that our reliance upon the mental health system for the basis of our recovery in dealing with quality of life is no longer needed. Instead we move back into society's realm of people, places and activities on our own two feet, healthy with supports in place that make our sustainability with functioning a reality.

Chapter 11

Values

Values are very important to recovery, and they are all too often misunderstood or mixed up with being morals; this they are not. Put simply, values are the things in life which we hold dear, They give meaning and purpose to our lives, and are the means by which we navigate our actions and behavior. Values are things like the desire to be loyal, to reach financial stability, success in a career, or health and well being among the many. We can lose track of our values during the onset of mental illness and this danger reflects in us by being symptomatic due to the fact that we are living against that which our internal make up and who we are yearns for us to be.

It is important in our roles as consumers to make sure that we know what things we value in life, or wish to value and bring about that change to have that value exist in our actions. Yes, our values do change over time, with regard to our age, stage of life we are in, and experiences. While some do change and we set out to incorporate those changes into our lives, there are still others that remain the same and have over time. It is vital to make sure that we do not wind up in a battle within ourselves by living out the actions and behavior which are non congruent to those which we hold as being important and valuable. Doing this can lead to further progression of our symptoms, or even a relapse when we are not being true to ourselves.

Of course the first thing to do is to assess your values that you have. Sometimes we get off track and forget to live by them, or even forget all about them as an entity, which leads to states of confusion. It is helpful to use the skill of journaling to assess your values and by writing them down get to learn more about who we are. The next step is to see how our actions and behavior clash with those values, then to make the appropriate changes in our life so that we live out who we are and the way we are, accepting this and communicating it with yourself in your own spirituality and the world. If there are new values that you wish to possess, then identifying them as well must occur as you explore the changes you wish to make in your life so that these values are carried out by yourself.

Only you can know what is right and best for yourself, and the journey of recovery is an individual one that needs to be tailored to your uniqueness. Sometimes the journey we have taken up to this point while doing battle with the symptoms of mental illness have put us into situations where we behaved adversely towards what our makeup is and the values we hold dear. This is where the pain from scarred emotions can come in. This is also just another opportunity to learn more about our triggers and how to process them, as well as the traumatic experience our spirit endured in going against our system of values. Regression is not an option here as we are moving forward in our recovery. Instead it is more of an opportunity to apply acceptance so that spirituality can grow in its strength as you in whichever way you choose to do so find that comfort and forgiveness in yourself, a forgiveness that comes to you through making amends to the people you may have harmed or to your own self if the action was harmful to you. Then you again with what we leaned through exploring our traumas shed it off and repeat the same mistake no more.

In turn when we set our system of values up in life and proceed to live by them, and being aware in our actions as we proceed with fulfilling the roles we desire and the roles we want to reestablish, we will find success. In this world it is often times seen as that the one who rushes to get to the top that is the winner, but in all actuality we see them fail. This failure is because they did not take the time out to assess their values as they proceeded with their destination in life. What is then left is a trail of heartache that will eventually catch up with them and have to be dealt with. As we activate our recovery our sense of developing our own value outlook on life and maintaining that will bring about empowerment amongst ourselves as we are now making the decisions towards gaining not only a foothold on recovery but on life.

When we get to this point in our recovery, we begin to see that we are growing, and with that growth comes responsibility. When assessing our values we see that that responsibility deals with ourselves and the actions that we take. Being conscious in the decisions and actions that we take takes determination, patience and hard work. It is not an easy process, especially when we have lived against our values battling within ourselves for whatever time we had been ill. Within this process is a pleasant side bar of being able to meticulously break down how we live our life, and by doing so we find ourselves involved more in the present state of being.

Another peer I had the pleasure to work with at one time came to a spot where he could analyze this in his recovery. He would openly share in group and individually with me and found himself stuck in trying to live down not only the values that other people had, which he thought he should bear, but also the inability to come to a conclusion about what things that he saw as having value.

When this peer and I sat down and shared, I saw a lot of myself within him as far as a recovery stage that I was in not long before I encounter. He did the things that the people who are assigned to see us through recovery advised him to do, and with due diligence. He unfortunately found himself unhappy and not enjoying the activities he was involved in. The reason being, and what he of his own accord came to realize, was that he was living his life by his own values, instead of by the values of others. He then set about to determine what his values were, for he was shocked when he did not know himself. This is not an uncommon phenomenon, for we as consumers often get lost in the pain and stress of managing our disease, get lost somewhere along the way about who we are as individuals, and values are a big makeup of who we are.

A way to help determine your values can be a simple as a top ten list. First you take this top ten list and format it by putting down all that you want to do, accomplish or see transpire in your life. These can also be used as goals, but then the real substance is when you further analyze these goals, and group them into categories of self determined values, brought about by this list. If you wrote down you wanted to make more money, then you have a value of wanting to be financially sound, if you have a goal to re-establish relationships with your family, then your value could be that you consider family life a high priority. Once all these values are determined, you keep them in order by not doing things which would cause damage to the structure of them. Sometimes unintentional damage is done, but this is the part where we must be aware and vigilant in living out our lives, which also promotes an active stance in our lives whereby we participate fully in the moment. We make wiser decisions and enjoy the benefits from those decisions.

Chapter 12

Awareness of One's Self

Self awareness is a part of our journey in our recovery that is vital to take at one point, a point where we have determined our values, made goals and objectives, and now it is time to look at our inner being and see who it is that we truly are. The way we view ourselves plays a part in our self esteem as well as the way we look at others. We as consumers should be in touch with how we feel about ourselves and how we feel about the outlook we have on how we participate in life. With self awareness comes the responsibility of being honest with ourselves so that we can come to a correct conclusion, with which we can make appropriate choices in our lives. It is by becoming self aware that we determine our strength, our weaknesses, and our wants and needs.

With our self esteem, and what we gain from the discovery of ourselves, we examine all of the strengths that we have as an individual. We look at where and what we excel in and find avenues to fit those strengths into our lives. When we explore our weakness as well we determine what the best plan of action is in order to transform that weakness into a strength. In doing this we know now in what ways we can best function.

When we are aware of our values and the things we hold dear, we can make better judgments in life with regard to living within the precepts of our make up. There is nothing more frustrating and nothing that brings about more pain that to live a life that is not in conjunction with who you are as an individual, and values are a big part of that. Living with that pain can cause an array of symptoms that aggravate our mental well being, and sometimes can cause a lack of functioning from their debilitating effects on us. They can also cause us to delve deeper into losing touch with who we are by determining to go against our values through behavior and actions that are contrary to them. This creates more emotions to deal with, which were created under the duress of living against your values.

One of the most important concepts of becoming self aware is learning to be honest with yourself. Sometimes we as consumers seem to overlook our weaknesses and not identify them, for example. When we do this we create an image within ourselves that when that subject does arise where these skills must be exhibited, we show that we cannot through failure. Failure is another feeling and emotion that we must take in, and if we bring this on by our own inability to be honest with ourselves then we are then bringing about the failure ourselves.

Being honest also means allowing the hidden traumas, hidden and kept secret by symptoms and avoidance, to come to light. Exploring our past is a big part of this continued concept of becoming self aware. It has been said that you never know who you are, if you forget where you have been. This holds true to us as mental health consumers as well. While this takes courage and patience, if we exhibit those attitudes and let the healing begin, it will continue with accepting the these experiences, and come to terms with what they make us today.

In incorporating these experiences along with their emotions we come to grips with the past so that we no longer have to be stuck living in it, with the symptoms of delusional fixations, depressions, and racing thoughts. Incorporation of these events into our self awareness leads us to where we want to be and where we aim to go. By shedding off these events after accepting them, and sometimes doing this with the communication skills we have begun to develop in our recovery when speaking with our therapeutic team members, we bring about a feeling of catharsis, a release of weeks, months or even years of trapped up energy, trapped by our own blocking techniques or disguised by our defense mechanisms.

Once we have become fully aware of all of these, and these are but a few, then we can better determine which way our life should take and which way we can live by in a more harmonious state. In our journey of recovery, remembering that everyone is unique is no more so than at this juncture. Only we can determine who we are, we have the keys that unlock those doors, and by practicing honesty with ourselves, allowing healing to occur, we build up our self esteem and become healthier people.

In my own recovery I came to a point where I became aware that I was indulging in my past with all the dysfunction that came along with the drug induced lifestyle of living that caused so many poor choices on my part. For me, I manipulated my conscious objections to the things I was participating in which were going against my values. While some values change over time, varying according to which stage you are in life and other factors, some stay the same and the goal to get back to living by those core values is imperative, as it was for me, by living against those and making excuses to my conscience in the form of delusions where I blamed God or even society; I was essentially in a war within my mind that I was unable to win without the acceptance of my past. Not only the acceptance of my past but the reconciliation of where in the form of spirituality I had to come to a sense of peace with my past so that I did not continue to get stuck in it. The next step that I had to take was to consistently reinforce the new way of thought and live according to my values not only through my actions but also in my thoughts.

Self awareness in these circumstances makes it to where you are able to examine your values, and when you come to a peace of the past conflict and start to live by those values that you battled with in the past, you also develop new ones in line with who you are as a person today. With all your experiences and knowledge of the life you led and the illness that once had control over our functioning, by being aware of who you are and who you want to become, you now have the horse by the reins. I was able to overcome my delusions one at a time, and as NA and other fellowships call this going through my individual spiritual awakenings, and seeing where they lead. The process of self awareness is one of the areas by which recovery from mental illness can be found and initiated.

The process of self awareness allows you to be aware of strengths and weaknesses. Strengths are a dynamic and important aspect of recovery, and in fact what many feel as the basis. This is certainly true as you become aware not only about what ways you were able to keep what sanity you may have had when going through those rough times, but also the strengths you have which have always been with you, in turn using all of these strengths to promote your recovery. With your weaknesses you find the areas where you might want to seek help. Weaknesses do not define you as weak, and it is in fact more or less a poor choice of word, but the areas where you could use more structure and build a firmer stance in the way you perceive and determine things.

I had a friend in life who was my peer. In our relationship we supported each other in our recovery. He found that he enjoyed his position in helping others very much. However he saw that his instability in being able to handle both family and work life got in the way of each other. He came to me and discussed this issue with me. He wanted to be involved with the revolution of sorts that was taking place in the mental health field with peer support and person centered treatment, but while he put all his energy into that, his mental health would suffer in his home life, and thus affect his family. He was heavy in heart with this decision and he was seeking support from me as a peer in determining the thing to do. The eventual decision was his and the one that he made was to leave the sometimes stressful work of serving others and tending to their needs and what is often the case overlooking his own. His weakness here was not that he could not handle the work load, because he did that fine. But the dilemma was actually in the fact that he poured himself whole heartedly into whatever he did, one hundred percent. When you are giving that much to something and there is no balance you find yourself not in a sense of whole life and whole health being.

When you examine the process of self awareness, it is important that we remember to examine all areas of our lives. When we focus just on one area and disregard the rest, we are in essence not allowing all areas of the scales to balance, leaving the chance for one of them to topple over the whole thing. This would require another rebuilding process and that is why the importance of spending a good amount of recovery oriented time in this area of self awareness is so important.

Chapter 13

Time Management

When looking at time management, it is funny to note that many people who are still under the power of the stigma of mental illness happen to believe that we do nothing with our time. While at some stages of our illness that can seem true by the standards of productivity, what we are doing is suffering the torments of the disease itself. From the lack of interests in things, which translates into low energy from inactivity, to the all encompassing racing thoughts and voices as well as other symptoms that we as mental health consumers have experienced, I would say that our time is indeed occupied.

When we as consumers have once found our motivators, set goals and objectives and worked our way through the recovery process thus far, and we find ourselves taking care of our needs and becoming involved in activities, it is here that time management plays a vital role in the concerns of our mental and overall health.

We are survivors of a disease and have fought to escape the hold it once had on us and we are coming closer to the time in our recovery where the management of our disease along with all of our efforts so far will be put to the test. Time management is the precursor to that, whereby we take another step in our recovery and place things in order so that the disarray of life which mental illness prowls on like fodder to the fire, does not engulf us as we maneuver to ascertain that responsibility and main goal of recovery.

Many of us have routines, or at least some point we did, and it is easiest and most natural to use that routine as the foundation of managing our time. We neglected our needs at one point, but now we find ourselves in a daily routine of managing our hygiene, and taking our medication for whatever health concern. For a while we might have been in isolation but now we have frequent engagements and appointments and responsibilities to tend to and be at. As all of these go with their ebb and flow of how we have begun to find a new meaning in life, a new measure by which we as consumers determine our own measurements of recovery and stabilization, a non linear one, which involves more than medication management and traditional clinical processes, many of these new pieces to our lives, or the restructuring of what once was, comes naturally in allowing time to run its course and not have the stress of trying to

meet deadlines and cram everything in. This natural method should be

encouraged, but we would be at fault if we did not know how to or take a

foothold in our recovery when it came to the time management of all of the

things which encompass themselves around us acting as an army defeating the

disease.

  Some tried and true tools of the trade have been appointment reminder books

and schedulers. Some of my fellow consumers have used daily routine logs,

especially when it comes to things like medicine or even hygiene. Alarm clocks,

alarms on watches, and even the old useful trick of tying a piece of yarn around

your finger as a reminder as you start out your day work are useful.

It is also indeed important to make sure that we utilize the recovery ideals that

help us manage our illness. Being in touch with our spirituality and taking time to

practice that which we hold evident in truth. Stress reduction sessions by which

we can do something as simple as deep breathing for a moment or two.

Journaling our thoughts and feelings for the day as well as keeping track of our symptom log, noting the time of the day and which emotion or expression or mood we are experiencing and its intensity. Taking the time in the day to reflect about our strengths and the resilience we have shown in coming this far, and the reminders of what our motivators are help us to grasp hold of the endurance needed for such a task as ours. Managing the tasks and finding the time to fit them in on a daily basis can be seen as vital to our recovery and mental health, while not becoming emotionally overdrawn as we do reflect, allowing thoughts and solutions to come and go, and not living a life bogged down by fear of missing a routine or two here and there. All the while remembering that life is meant to be lived, and that the level and titration by which your recovery tasks are needed, will be decided by you, the consumer, whose own unique journey of recovery must suit them.

In my own life, I have many medical complications along with having the diagnosis of schizo affective disorder. This of course is not uncommon as it is estimated that people with mental illness have a 25 year shorter life span that someone without, and much of that statistic is do to the multiple diagnoses we are faced with. Whether it be from neglecting our needs at a point, or the construct of a side effect of medication meant to help manage our disease, some of us find ourselves bogged down at times by the onslaught of the medical illnesses, yet there is hope. The hope is in this time management. Like everything else in life our health both physical and mental has to be managed. In the society we live in today, we rely on a host of different doctors with the idea that our family practice doctor will manage all of the symptoms, but it is up to us to manage the treatment.

When I was diagnosed with diabetes, I wasn't exactly sure what it was. I was more than certain that it was from the obesity caused by being on neuroleptics, and I was already inundated with other medical issues besides managing my mental health. So I did what came naturally to a person who feels overwhelmed and like an ostrich stuck my head in a hole and hoped I wouldn't have to deal with it. Unfortunately this wasn't the case for me and I would have to eventually deal with it, being forced to take my blood sugar every day and watch my diet, due to natural consequences of yet another illness caused by diabetes which was gastrointestinal, and that was the kick in the rear that I needed to take that part of my health more seriously and not ignore it any more. I started to manage it and saw the results quite quickly.

There is a hero I often use as an illustration of how they used a specific technique and molded it to fit their own recovery, in the hope that it serves as an inspiration to others as it does to me, that recovery is possible and we can learn from one another. I came across her while serving on the act team at a local clinic in my home town. She had a way about her, she walked upright, very proud of her accomplishments, which she had the right to be. She did not let the stigma of mental illness affect her in any way, but was forthcoming to anyone who asked her about the topic and did so with a so what type of attitude. She was an inspiration to me and a fellow peer who ran groups at the clinic.

She had a history of trauma in her life which she revealed to me, but I don't think that is worthwhile looking into or disclosing. Rather, I see the traits which she had which made her the individual she was, and a lot of keeping herself above the waters that can sometime drown us into becoming symptomatic and regressing in our recovery, she did so with organization and a strict time management routine making you believe she could run a fortune five hundred company, which in fact she most likely could. Not only was she a peer who ran groups, but she also maintained a part time job outside of that work in real estate as well as raised one of her own grandchildren. Even with him she did amazing things, acting upon his star quality and getting him involved with magazines and modeling as well as acting.

What a busy life she had, but to her it was one of fulfillment. She didn't miss a beat. When it came to her health one thing about her which I learned and gained insight from was that she was not afraid to tell someone no. We often times get ourselves into situations where we are afraid to do what is right and best for our own health and well being by wanting to be a service to others and thus taking on more than we can handle. With her she knew her limits, yet she felt she had none; saying no was just a choice, not a fault, but a decision, and in that decision doing what was best for her overall goal of recovery.

Remembering to manage our time and the events which are constructed around it is vital to recovery, with our natural ability to focus our energy on those that come without effort and then adding to that which requires a reminder on our part. Taking every aspect of our lives seriously at the time it is dealt and not putting if off with a sense of procrastination and knowing when to say no to someone so as not to over exert yourself are all time management traits and tools that we as consumers should utilize in our journey of recovery. It will bring about that goal of recovery in the time that it is meant to be fulfilled and with an easier transition than the struggles of being unorganized and the stress which that would bring along the way. Be diligent in your recovery, take the time to enjoy life as you move through it, and the time to rejuvenate yourself as well.

Chapter 14

Emotions

Emotions and processing them is a huge part of being mentally healthy. There are different types of emotions and although some have been labeled as bad emotions, all emotions are vital to the existence of human beings. Emotions are one of the things that sets us apart from other living creatures in the full array of the ones that we are at liberty to express. The first step is knowing all the different types of emotions so that you are aware of what you are experiencing. There is no greater fear, especially when a consumer of mental health services and all the symptoms that come along with being labeled as such than not knowing or being able to explain what you are feeling or experiencing. While I can only offer a few in the limited space I have in this book as the topic is so large but important enough for recovery and by which the way I gained my own recovery and witnessed others find theirs, just like when we in our process of recovery utilizing this book educated ourselves in our illness, so too should we educate ourselves on emotions and the different types.

Some have said that there are god emotions and bad. This type of thinking can be misleading, but rather look at emotions as either comfort or discomfort when experiencing them. This first step while still a marginal basis by which to categorize them is important as we do divide them into ones which bring us different emotional feelings. Things like joy, happiness, and laughter bring us comfort. Other emotions such as anger, fear, and frustration bring us discomfort. The important part of bringing these all in the make up of who you are as an individual is not in fending off the ones you feel discomfort with, for they will come again, but rather knowing how to process them. The same holds true for the emotions which are known to bring us comfort, learning and knowing how to produce those feelings as well as have control over them in the process of them so that we don't go overboard as some may lead to questionable behavior.

In this day and age we have been taught to hide our emotions, not let anyone in, guard our hearts from the mistrust that had become our generation's key component of functioning. We are consumers of an illness which engulfs itself along things like emotions, memories, thoughts, and feelings, that make up the person we are and define the struggles that we have, and serve as clues as to how to better reach our ultimate goal of recovery where all of these facets of life are seen on an orderly position by ourselves and one which we are content with and able to manage.

After we have identified the different types of emotions and have ourselves grounded about the way it makes us feel individually, then comes the healing by which we learn how to process them. Anger, a considerably uncomfortable emotion, is not necessarily a bad one, nor one which we should avoid ourselves from embracing if it does indeed come. Taking anger as an example, the key is to identify the feeling, find the etiology or source of where it had come from, and if need be process it in a manner that is healthy and beneficial to us in our mental and emotional well being. Often times emotions are observable through our actions and behavior, and many times that is why we see many of our fellow consumers being force medicated in hospitals, one of those being me at one time in my life, due to the inability to control or rather process my feeling of anger and lash out at anyone who was in my vicinity.

The better thing to do is to educate ourselves again on how to control these emotions. Some tools are using exercise to relieve the stress from it in it those moments of high intensity to work off the steam which can build to more erratic behavior. It is also an opportunity to determine the source of the anger and come to resolutions and compromise. Compromise is another tool, and it is important to remember our step of acceptance of things whereby we are in control, not the trigger that is causing the discomfort.

The same holds true for those emotions that bring about feelings of happiness, joy and laughter. The key to those most of the time is that we have no doubt about where the etiology or source of those emotions are coming from. They are not blocked by the poor processing that we often times see as consumers with the discomfort emotions which lead to a display of our emotions and the inability to logically and consciously define the problem and come with a solution to it. These comfort feelings, when they come, do just that, bring comfort. It is helpful to us as consumers as we undergo this transformation from being bogged down by symptoms, to create these comfort emotions sometimes for ourselves. We can do that by entertaining our minds with video games, movies, and books that we enjoy. Being involved in activities that we find meaning in is not only one of these steps but also a source of happiness. We get these feeling when we reflect and see that we have accomplished a goal or objective, it gives us pride in what we have accomplished, and it builds our self esteem as we are aware of who we are and how far we have come and what we have overcome.

The biggest mishap of all which we as consumers most certainly should avoid and I on a constant basis remind myself to practice, is not to bottle up our feelings and emotions. In doing that healing cannot occur, and in fact damage can be done which can possibly resurface along down the road of recovery and act as a speed bump and stall us. Another thing that can occur if we hold these feelings and emotions inside and do not allow time for processing is that our behavior can start to become out of control, we burn bridges that we have developed with others, and we can begin to create a look of poor self esteem with regard to ourselves.

A friend and peer of mine also had a diagnosis of mental illness, and this was early on in my first stage of being diagnosed, and now I can look back on it with a different view of how she was able to overcome and handle her daily life. Not only was she battling a mental illness, but she like many of our peers had problems with marriage, relationships and finances. She was a hard worker and was employed at the same place where I was and that was how I came to know her.

In looking back I saw how she grew, from moments of being so downtrodden that she would break down and cry right there at work and have to take some time for herself which wasn't a good thing in a fast paced work environment that we were in, but the staff were all understanding as I was and helped her through. She had held many things in and in an unconscious effort isolated herself from almost everyone and anyone that could bring meaning into her life or serve as a system

of support. We sometimes find that emotions are brought on by our interactions

with others and without any interaction we are left to not grow and wallow in the

past mistakes where the hurt just continues and no resolution is seen.

There is where I first understood the meaning not only of being a friend but being

a supportive peer, one who was there to help with a heart of understanding and

empathy of the things that she had gone through. It was not a physical or

romantic relationship we had but rather one of emotional support. By that

emotional support we were able to have new emotions come into existence

through the memories that we made and the resolutions to old problems that we

kept boiling up inside.

We as we go through our recovery journey, see that not only are we people of

courage and strength and vitality, by which we continue on towards our main goal

of recovery for ourselves, but we are also a beacon to others. As we follow the

examples of recovery, by whatever means you find it works best for you, be it this

book, or another, or a peer involved group, in growing we share, and through

sharing we grow, giving to each other the spirit of hope which is one of the first

we started out with. In having no home, we had to believe that there was hope,

and find reasons to go on, and take on the responsibility of recovery. Now giving back to others that hope brings us to the next phase in our journey and that is how we manage our recovery as we grow and build upon it.

Taking a look at a few of the underfunded facilities and the conditions consumers must bear while attempting to recover from an episode of psychosis, depression or another label would break down even the hardest heart to tears These conditions, while not the norm across the nation, leaves many consumers still far away from the goal of recovery.

MANAGE

In this third phase of recovery we focus on the management of all the recovery practices we have partaken in. We take an investigation of our behavior and make sure that we have control over them and are able to recognize when they are peeking out at us and in need of attention.

We focus on in this phase of recovery all of our needs, making sure that our basic needs are met as well as those of our emotional well being are considered. The nurturing of those needs which we have, including the spiritual ones which can promote well being in recovery, are examined.

We will take a look at the growth process we have undergone as well as reflecting on all that which we have accomplished in our recovery and in our lives. Perhaps one of the most significant points of recovery are made here in the concept of empowerment and how we as consumers should be engaged actively making decisions in our lives and our treatment.

Chapter 15

Managing Behavior

In life the mental health system as it stands now judges our progress by our actions and behavior. This can be quite a scary thought to some of us consumers who have seen the system of care at its worst.

It is also of importance to look at recovery as a responsibility. We as consumers have been known to put ourselves in dangerous situations where our actions take us. Seeking help through illicit drugs and self medicating, or comfort in the form of a prostitute while struggling with the hypersexual urges that accompany mental illness. We know of peers that have come to be known as cutters or rather use self harm as a way of relief of symptoms. Trouble with the law is not unheard of, where tempers flare and in our manic state we sometimes find ourselves acting as a superhuman. This is the result of television news as survivors of or even victims of death by stun guns from the police whose training may or may not be up to date on how to serve a person with a mental illness.

Perhaps the most important part of learning to manage our behavior in its most outlandish forms is the responsibility that we have to society to firstly not cause our illness to harm others I am a believer that we as individuals are responsible for our actions and how we are judged is left to the courts system of fair justice. However, this shows the even more importance of why we as consumers especially at this stage of recovery where we are here by managing our recovery, take on the responsibility of managing our own behavior as well as being aware of any peers that we come across along the way, looking out for the best interest of all.

We have looked at many aspects of recovery, one of those being values. As we have determined our values; it is important that we not lose sight of them, for here is where they can come in handy as a judge of sorts as to how we are living according to how our minds makeup of central belief is concerned. Do we do things that go against what we believe, are we making decisions that are contrary to our objectives and goals? These are some of the hidden aspects of behavior modification that we can undertake, but there still remain the ones that are visible, to us as consumers, and to our supporters, as well as therapeutic team members.

There can be behavior such as slowly losing interest in the things we care about. Sleeping more than usual or spending more money than we would normal undertake on expenditures, the basics of symptom management. We all know that medicine is the cure for mental illness, and so it is down to us to take steps towards reinforcing the medicated effects it you take them, or reevaluation of your natural alternative to recovery when these symptoms arrive. It is through symptoms many times that our behaviors are brought to being, so it can be said that they are the precursor to our actions when looking at mental health with that pair of eyes.

Remembering our tools of symptom log books, and doing a fresh new reflection at times on how we are doing should be encouraged in us. Having confidantes and close friends or other peers that know our actions and behavior when we are not at are best, so that they can sound an alarm bell to us and for us, before further damage to our recovery is done. It would be nice if recovery's journey came with the grace of never falling back into old habits or old symptoms arising, but that is not guaranteed and we should always be mindful, especially during times of stress, or when we are having trouble with triggers or memories brought about by coincident in the present time of our recovery.

I know that this is not the best of topics to discuss and doesn't produce that great productive 'I can do this' feeling of recovery that we have come to know in our journey, but we are more mature now as we go on our way and should look at things now as a test of perseverance once again, holding fast to the fact that we have shown that in the resilient way we have come in our recovery thus far. But I feel it important also because it is a reality and sometimes a dark reality of how sometimes we can become so very ill and bad things can happen, not intentionally by us but through our disease's control over us. It reminds me of a consumer who I was serving while on the act team at a clinic. The morning that she was assigned to the clinic coming out of one of the state hospitals there was a big meeting at the clinic regarding reporters and the like as it was a very high profile client.

Without naming the client or having any damage done other than to say that this client's action before coming to the community clinic resulted in death, I wasn't sure how I would handle this, it was new to me at my point of recovery but the clinic thought I would understand the person and be best suited for the task of being the case manager as I have a mental illness. In working with this person, I know that they wanted life to go on for them as well, without the media, without the intervention of caseworkers coming to their home causing a stir. However, I found that it should have been more important even here with this person about the role we have in the responsibility of our recovery as to not to put ourselves into situations where we can be triggered at a time we might not be ready, or to move too fast without fully grasping every aspect or even skipping an important part of recovery. I disagreed with a lot of what this consumer was doing in their recovery plans and eventually asked to be taken off as their caseworker.

Here at this point in our recovery journey, taking a look and reflecting upon what our behavior once was and where we are now is somewhat of a wake up call to the seriousness of the disease and the importance of continuing to practice the modules of recovery.

Chapter 16

Attentiveness to our Needs

and

Alternative Methods of Care

Recognizing what our needs are, emotionally, socially, and physically, and being attentive to them is an all important aspect of the care we give ourselves in terms of maintaining a healthy mental health outlook. With all the responsibilities in life that we already have in place along with the the one which requires sometimes a more in depth look and greater attention, that being our mental health, our own needs can be overlooked sometimes as we pay more attention to the needs of our illness and not our innate needs. We have needs of being spiritual, to have accomplishment be seen in our lives, and many other of the plethora of emotional and humanistic things which in our society we seek to attain. So, as consumers, it is helpful to make note of this and live life in the moment taking care of those needs, both physical and mental, pursuing recovery while maintaining life's everyday functioning.

We see that we have emotional needs, as in the activate your recovery series, we examined the types and the healthy ways in which to process them. We are also aware that we have dreams and aspirations, built on hopes and goals when we looked into recovery in motion and started our journey keeping the wheels of recovery in motion and not getting stuck in what I like to call the doldrums. We have the need to be symptom free and seek out healing for our traumas and learn how to manage the triggers that present themselves to us in life, all of these along with managing them in the time we have on this earth to find our fulfillment in the type of recovery which we as consumers individually seek, are all in the process of being attentive to our needs. We are starting to see that non linear approach examined here in these recovery is motion series guides, first presented and suggested towards a module of recovery by fellow consumers, people in their support system, and therapeutic guides, then outlined and set forth in SAMHSA principles towards reaching recovery. An approach that is holistic, and osteopathic medically treating the illness as it pertains to all avenues of our lives. We also know as Maslow stated in his pyramid of needs, that everyone in this world, including us as consumers, need the basic needs as well. Things such as shelter, clothing, food, all those are among our absolute needs, and in some cases for us as consumers and for our fellow peers we see a need for assistance and aid in that department. Hopefully after battling a disease like no other, the one we refer to generically as a mental illness, we gather our strengths in recovery, building upon our hopes, setting out goals, resurrecting our time managing skills, and moving on to sustain these needs by our own measures.

I was once told that recovery cannot happen until these are all in place, and that saddened me in the way that those whom I worked with from time to time in the mental health system where I was in the position as a peer provider, put as I saw it, limits upon my fellow consumers, preventing recovery from taking place because the consumers they were serving were lacking these things. Then I found someone who agreed with me, a fellow consumer and peer provider, a veteran of America's armed forces, who shared his story with me about his journey of recovery. He had lost his home, his position of employment, and the little he did have in government aid he spent on a daily alcohol habit. However this peer of mine found his recovery with a therapeutic guide who took upon themselves to do all of the psychosocial rehabilitation steps together, instead of taking it bit by bit. With all of these things in motion for him as he lived at a homeless shelter for a period of time, he found recovery while at the same time attending to his physical needs.

What this allowed him to do was grow. Many of us consumers are told in essence to stop life as we try to recover, a philosophy, that of recovery, that not too long ago was thought impossible by many members of the psychiatric community. When we as consumers are allowed these avenues of participation we grow in not only our recovery but in life as individuals along with everyone else in the world who participate in life's daily living routine. This is where I feel the mental health system as we know it does the most damage to us in the form of reinforcing that stigma of a mental health patient, treating us while we work in recovery as a person who is lost completely, and has no chance at all for mental health recovery, especially if the functioning that a consumer once had has led them to the dire straits such as homelessness and isolation from society itself. When we are separated from that of an individual who is allowed to grow in life while they go through their own unique difficulties, then we are thus looked at as different, not allowed to grow and stigmatized.

I am not as a fellow consumer up to date with all of the different avenues of recovery that are termed as alternatives. I live my recovery by the way I have envisioned my goals and aspirations to be. I manage my symptoms through what most would say are traditional methods, with some fluctuations here and there. But I do as part of this recovery series guide, and as a person who believes that all avenues to recovery and knowledge should be given, make sure that that exists here. I myself work with massage therapy and chiropractic, and other therapies, incorporating exercise and diet into my life as a means of maintain my recovery. Those of my fellow consumers who search should not be afraid to search these avenues as well. There is a conference in the U.S. with the title alternatives of which I will attend my first one which is held yearly this upcoming 2012. Everyone's needs are unique and derived out of their own personal values and experiences. With this in mind attentiveness to our own needs sometimes means looking outside the box. However, I have found that looking outside the box, often times I come across things that are already in the box, and am able to adapt them to my own needs as a person. Not every little smidgen of suggestion needs to be followed like an unbreakable rule with dire consequences, but having a guide is helpful and allows you to grow with the use of it as a person who takes knowledge and applies it to their own life as it will work for them.

At this point in the recovery is motion series, it is a good point to break and examine what it is we are all trying to accomplish. Recovery most certainly is one of the goals for each consumer, or the maintaining of recovery; one has found this is helpful for as well. As we look at attentiveness to one's needs, we can ask ourselves what were those needs we had which we longed for relief from? The symptoms of mental illness in whatever form it presents itself and the relief from those symptoms that once may have had us hunkering down in life, and through this recovery is motion series, utilizing a holistic type of a non linear approach where you yourself my fellow consumer has been informed, hopefully inspired by some of the other consumers whose successes I share with you have inspired me, and an all encompassing approach to knowledge about recovery modules to use in your journey, all the while hopefully healing your traumas, processing your emotions, and controlling your triggers. I could have written and have written about depression's causes and symptoms, the sources of delusions and thought insertion, and my own little pet project of examination of foilie de deuxs and their existence amongst mental health consumers inside the confined walls of the hospital, but I prefer to keep recovery goal oriented, positive, solution based, and practical, while also incorporating spiritual growth, building upon strengths, nurturing our hopes, and through all this bringing empowerment to the consumer, or individual seeking recovery. Empowerment could be viewed as the finished bi product of recovery, whereby we gain control of our own lives which had once been under the control of this dreadful disease of mental illness and the symptoms which came along with it.

I am reminded of a friend, and fellow peer, who I witnessed recovery take place throughout him in many areas. He finally reached a point where he told me that he was going to go to school and then move to Florida so that he could enjoy the beach while he made a living. He said he had worked on managing his recovery for a long time now, and that it has given him a sense of empowerment, of control over the decisions he was able to make for himself, whether small or big in nature. In all of it he said, that if he would not have managed his recovery while he was engaged in it, then he would have never been able to benefit from the work he had put into it. So as we look at important aspects in this series of managing our recovery, let's stay focused on the topics shared, along with all that we have learned and gained along the way in our own unique approach to transcending, with these guiding topics, knowing that we are now invested in and taking on the responsibility of recovery.

Chapter 17

Nurturing Our Recovery

As a father of 6 years now, I have learned in that manner much patience, love, frustration, and joy goes into nurturing a living human being. Many of you my fellow consumers have gone through the parenting process as well while either wrestling with a mental illness, or throughout different phases of your own recovery. Others have nurtured children, projects, or even other family members along the way. Without consistent nurturing of something, we can let what we are trying to nurture feel neglected, or that person or thing we are nurturing become more independent in itself, taking a life of its own.

The same holds true when we as consumers need to be prepared and responsible in managing our recovery and taking time to nurture the things that we have worked on. All we have undertaken from learning to express emotions, learning to be content and accepting of things, and being motivated by our desires, and applying that by practicing the management of our behavior. When we don't do this, especially with a disease unlike any other, that of mental illness, it can truly make us feel neglected, or the disease itself can take on a life of its own, and lead us down a path of further injury in our recovery process.

In examining how to nurture our recovery, it is best be looked at as a method of practice. When we practice at things, in all of life's makeup of things, we become better, more apt to the challenge of whatever it is we are fixated on while applying ourselves to master it. Practice can mean such things, in regards to recovery, as formulation of new daily affirmations to go along with your daily routine. I have known peers that have made a game of it and tied it into their practice of spirituality and value based way of living life whereby they use a different one each week or even day, to eventually live and master that so that it is firmly placed in their memory bank to rely on in times of need. This like many other modules we as consumers can practice leads us to formulating inside our minds, creating a backlog of coping skills that we can lean on in times of crisis or when we are faced with triggers. Instead of the defense mechanism we often undertook led by our mental illness of allowing symptoms to be that way of coping, we now with assuredness of a practiced individualized plan, choose from those modules of defense when life's stressors get the best of us.

Stress is a huge topic in mental illness, and one that most certainly needs attention given to. As we nurture our recovery we also nurture ourselves in ways that promote healthy stressful releases. I get made fun of often times, as I am a bigger man, beard and all, thought of as a man's man by some, and when we are in group or I am attending a conference and the question arises about what we do for stress, I always answer with take a bubble bath. Now all joking aside, that form of relief is actually a good one as the steam rises in the hot water filled tub and fills the room, sweating out the impurities in your system, and this is just one idea, and an easy one of which is ready available to most. Others may find that reading a book in a quiet setting, or even taking a kick boxing class releases built up tension, but whatever the routinely practiced event, its nurturing value is essential to our recovery in more ways than one.

We know that it produces relief from stress, but it is also nurturing in that it builds upon what we have examined in this recovery is motion series an awareness of one's self. We come to see what makes us comfortable when we are stressed or agitated, and we come to find an identity behind what we as human beings enjoy. Nurturing in this way gives us a foundation upon which we can build, finding similar activities along the way. In this upcoming year I will be applying for my license in chemical dependency counseling and I have studied it throughout my years of schooling, not to mention being a friend of the bill in working the twelve steps and my participation in NA. One thing I have learned throughout that, and one thing that I find very common amongst those of us who call ourselves consumers, peers, peer providers or even survivors, is that when we have such things as a memory of a delusion that has spent years racing through our minds, it has formulated itself into an existence within ourselves that in order to be disregarded must be replaced by something else in life that we do or conceive in thought. It is the same with all the different types of symptoms accompanying mental illness, as it is true in algebra and mathematics what you do to one side you must always to to the other. It's a step in replacement, similar to that of why they say there is no cure for addiction, that addicts learn to live day by day and replace that which they used to do with positive productive life activities, surrounding themselves with other addicts who have had similar experiences. It is also important to note that while addicts have found such a fellowship we to have a similar one where we look to nurture ourselves and our recovery in the form of peer support and peer support groups and activities. I have participated in peer support groups both as a facilitator and a participating member seeking assurance and help through the strengths of others. This process is like no other and it has now climbed its way, in the U.S., into our mental health system and while there are still barriers in place, input from consumers is now being looked at in a positive manner as true meaningful avenues in which to find recovery.

Another means of nurturing our recovery is by involvement in activities, which is the first of the recovery topics discussed in this manual. It was placed there specifically for the purpose of making sure that the consumer who is seeking out recovery is made aware of groups out there that provide support and the importance of leaning upon those groups so as to build a stronger system of support as we as consumers make our way down this sometimes rocky road of recovery.

Where we are now seeking out to manage our recovery, we see the true work not only in the reflection of what we have done thus far towards our recovery, but what it takes to continuously manage our recovery. It is an ongoing process, one without a finish line. Yes, there are points and moments in which we find joy and accomplishment, and places where we find our objectives met and emotional health restored. Hopefully as well in working these series of workbooks, symptoms have gone astray and living life is now done on your own terms, conquering the once stronghold form of a defense system we had leaned on to help manage our functioning in life and our processing of events which came in the form of symptom display from a mental illness, and now leaning on these given practices for support . In order for this to continue we look at the practice involved and the management of all things including nurturing our own needs where we are responsibly working our recovery as it is in motion and not letting

that inertia come to a halt.

Chapter 18

Answering Spiritual Needs

There are many ways to practice spirituality as noted, and for the purposes of this book we will examine the basic ones which are used by many, the first one being meditation. Meditation does not have to refer to some type of religious practice, some people often call it prayer and reflection. In using it for this purpose of reflection, I have found it as well as many of my peers helpful in many ways. One of those ways in which it is helpful is by allowing thoughts to come and go in a natural way while the investigation of your inner voice speaks to you in whatever event, emotion or other life activity occurred that day. This is most well suited to be done in an environment where calmness safety and quiet can be found. Many practice by deep breathing and concentration on certain thoughts such as a daily inspiration repeated over and over in your mind.

Spirituality as we know it does exist on a realistic plane as we feel its effects on the levels of stress we endure, the moments of peace we have, and the assuredness that we as with others who practice their spirituality exist in this community as givers and takers and participators in life. In practicing it on a realistic plane if you will, that being one of substance where actions can be seen, we can do things such as look out for our fellow human being with acts of kindness, patience, and good will. We have all heard of the golden rule do unto others and it is a positive one to live by, and one which will most likely reduce the amount of stress and anxiety along with the other types of nuances which come with the disease of mental illness.

I am going to make this statement, and it is my hope that I am not looked at by my fellow peers as one who does not want to break free from a tradition of addictions, as I do consider myself an addict, but also a consumer/survivor, but it is my own belief that we as a group of unique people who are making leaps and bounds into participatory inclusion into our own care, follow some of the guidelines set forth by those first self help help groups and pioneers in the world of addictions which is often times cross-referenced. One of those guidelines which I feel the absence of from our main goal of recovery is that of the belief in a higher power. Again everyone's spiritual journey in life is one that they must make on their own. I have my own which may or may not be revealed by the symptoms I have shared in this self help type recovery manual, and without that basic foundation it can cause many roadblocks for future healing to occur. One of those roadblocks being inclusion into society, and the use of natural resources of

recovery termed so by psych rehab professionals, by participating in social groups

and fellowships of such things as churches and synagogues and temples.

The other road block which can present is at the very beginning of recovery where

we as consumers can have at the onset a hope given to us to start off with when

at times all hope is considered lost. This is where motivation starts, what the

counselors call pre contemplation and contemplation of the decision to take on

the responsibility of recovery, and the outlook of hope is what we find as one of

those key ingredients in the start and making sure recovery is in motion.

One final point to make is that in a world where it seems like nobody cares,

especially if that world is viewed by the eyes of a consumer of mental health

services, a belief in some type of higher power is comforting to those of us looking

for rest from the weary war of the mind, and uplifting as we see others that have

embraced it among our ranks.

Spirituality can also for consumers be a a strong rock by which to focus on where

we can give explanations to the troublesome events, emotional scars and altered

moods that we often times have. In practicing the different aspects of spirituality

and starting to manage it as well we as consumers will find a more significant

growth when applying it to all the topics of recovery that we have in these series covered thus far. We might, some of us, even have what in NA and other fellowships call a spiritual awakening.

I have two stories of such to share about consumers, who have come to me inquiring about spiritual advice, both of them at opposite spectrums of outcomes. The first consumer I met about half into my long journey of ongoing recovery at a time where I was working as a qualified mental health para professional. He was put on my caseload of consumers whom I have had the pleasure to serve and had a diagnosis of schizo affective disorder dually diagnosed with chemical dependency. He was living in a boarding house, one which is well maintained and one which I hope I have the opportunity to share with you if the topic permits in the series where once again we revisit living arrangements. He was in that what they call the pre-contemplation stage, moving back and forth from using and staying clean and his habit was disrupting his mental illness as he continued to use.

The topic of spirituality came up when he asked me about certain aspects of a religion, one which if I were to reveal to him we had common ground on. I was fairly knew to the world of mental health and working for a state funded mental health clinic, and I was reluctant to go forward on the subject without first consulting my supervisor. I told them the situation and how he was wanting me to visit with him on the subject where he was hoping someone with a similar background could share from a peer point of view so that he could come to a conclusion. The answer to me from my supervisor was that I was not to go anywhere near that subject with him. I did the best I could and gave him a handout on the matter, and with him noticing avoidance from me saw yet another person not willing to walk with him in his recovery, and wound up back on the streets living the life of a drug using consumer with criminal activities surrounding him amongst the friends he had made. Needless to say the stance that many of us as consumers and the mental health system have taken as a whole until recently regarding the inclusion of spirituality on concepts integrated into recovery from a mental illness, while at that time there was none, left another consumer sadly misinformed, alienated, and further distraught.

The next consumer I met with while working specifically as a peer support specialist. He had come to many meetings and is the same individual who we examined a glimpse of into his recovery when we covered spirituality early on in this recovery is motion series. Both of us have had almost identical delusional creativeness about our illness and in its use as a defense mechanism, and after building that bound of trust which Adler so remarkably makes clear is a necessary step in the therapeutic process, and in life and relationships in general, he was able to reveal to me his hidden thoughts that he had kept in with fear, left inside tormenting him the whole tenure of his time with poor mental health, until he was able to connect with another peer and find that it is a common misconception and learn ways of how to handle such thoughts that would benefit him in his own spiritual walk, as well as in his own recovery.

For me, spirituality has played a vital role in my recovery. From the onset of my decline from the use of drugs and the decision to enter into a rehabilitation program fourteen years ago, I sought out answers to my traumas, emotional upheavals, and reasons to keep trekking on life's journey. Along the way it was twisted in the mire of mental illness symptoms and became a stumbling block for me as well as my strength and inspiration, and then later a healing touch was brought into it where I was able to recognize myself in what I believed and no longer lived in fear of the unknown or uncertainty.

I hope that all can find their spirituality in the way which it comes to them, and that it can be managed in your recovery as a vital tool, with its aid helping gain a foothold on dreams and aspirations while learning to live in the moment, and process you feelings, organize your thoughts, and conquer your moods.

Chapter 19

Growth and Reflection

One of the intentions of this book, while of course being to aid my fellow

consumer in reaching their coal of recovery, one in which they measure its

success in their own terms, I have also tried my best to incorporate all the behind

the scenes knowledge if you will of what I have witnessed, learned and

participated in while working in the mental health field in different positions for

over five years now. That knowledge along with my knowledge from studying

rehabilitation in a scholastic setting, and the knowledge base I have as a

consumer of services for over fourteen years, I, in this series, wanted to make

sure that that knowledge and information was not kept hidden from those in

search of their own recovery. That knowledge is power and with it we as

consumers can build upon it and formulate our own type of recovery plan which

comes naturally with participating in these readings and handouts, as they are

geared with the consumer's choice in mind.

This is the growth which I hope that the consumers and supporters of consumers who take on the responsibility of recovery by utilizing this series will be motivated to seek, accepting of it, manage it as it grows and eventually benefit from it and reap life's rewards. Growth and reflection upon that growth is a rewarding and all encompassing task that we take on while in this management phase of recovery. We look back and practice the tools and ideas that each one of you as consumers has developed in their journey of recovery, and we stay motivated to keep up this responsibility through the inspirational stories and the insightful examination of other consumers and situations they have been in during times of their recovery where I have had the privilege to cross paths with them. Most importantly however is that the reflection of each and every consumer who utilizes this series in their recovery will gain a since of accomplishment, joy, and confidence in the journey they have undertaken.

Practicality in recovery is essential and a concept I have tried my best to incorporate in this series as well. Useful guidelines, and tools and coping strategies of how to work recovery, so that it in turn works for you, have been successful for me in my own journey of recovery and in others whom I have seem blossom like a compressed lump of coal being formed through the pressures of a debilitating disease, and through the unique type of people that we are, in our strength and resiliency turned into beautiful priceless diamonds.

One of those tools that I have found useful when modeling the guideline of growth and reflection is the infamous journal, which every consumer has been suggested by others into putting to use at sometime or another in their recovery, and for good reason. I myself when starting out my journal in looking back see it go from writing down what the weather was that day and how exhausted I felt, to pages upon pages of goals, accomplishments in meeting those goals, and my personal thoughts of how I have grown as a person in my emotions, accepting myself for who I was and others for who they are, and how my life had become filled with numerous involvements in different activities which have found their way into my life through breaking out of my shell from the onset and not allowing the stigma nor the symptoms tell me how my life was going to turn out to be. When you journal which I hope you have practiced and set aside time to manage that task from the beginning, you will most likely find the value in it as I have and others who have shared their success with me in the use of this tool. It is a show of history like none other, the history of yourself, and the defeat of the villain which used to consume you. It will be upon reading a roller coaster of ups and downs, joyous occasions as well as trying tasks you have undertaken, and it will give you insight into discovery of yourself and how you can utilize that and all the other knowledge you have gained to manage your recovery and to progress in life with the firm affirmation that you are a person who is very self aware of who you are, and have no limits by which fear can stall you in your many different escapades in life. Write in it as often as you can, take time with it, and review it on a basis which you feel comfortable in your own recovery.

The same serves true for those old symptom logs and at times you will know in your recovery when and when not to use them as the need arises, hopefully as a consumer engaged in managing their recovery and concerned with the management of their own behavior as well.

Coming from a consumer who has gone in and out of the workforce from time to time, those pay check stubs that have been lying around in your desk, or that notice of final disability payment are encouraging and can bring back moments of butterflies in the stomach feelings. Projects which you have started and completed during this time, sons and daughters who you have now had better relations with and more joyful occasions with, as well as other family members, co-workers and friends whose bridges you thought were once burned, recollection of these will build more avenues of motivation so as to not digress, and thankfulnesses in your spirit that you have found the strength within yourself to overcome.

I myself upon taking out time for reflection, have visited different clinics where I use to work or have been a consumer receiving services from at one time. Engaging with the doctors and other staff that were there assisting you at a time when you felt you needed it, and sharing with them how you have found recovery and what it means to you, proving to others that recovery is possible, while at the same time thanking them for what they were able to do for you during your time of need. This is also helpful to a consumer who has developed a passion like many of us do that go through the recovery process to become part of a care team as a peer provider in some array of function in the mental health system at a position, and these visitations can open doors to positions in specific clinics, research opportunities, and sometimes even speaker occasions for those interested in learning about recovery.

I have just recently been given the opportunity, through this type of networking, an opportunity which I have accepted and am weighed down with a heavy heart as far as the importance of its fruition. It was from an old caseworker who aided me in my recovery, had seen me at my worst, and then found me walking through the same doors she did as a peer specialist as a co-worker. In speaking with her about my recovery - all the steps I have taken and what I have accomplished - she suggested my services to the national institute of mental health here in the U.S.. The main goal of this program is reaching out to grade schoolers at around the age of eleven and twelve and speaking with them, trying to put an end to the stigma involved with having a mental illness, education and understanding, and prevention.

This takes me to my next point about growth and reflection. I had an opportunity another time to lead on a similar cause for a non profit organization. At that time I was ailing in my health and symptomatic although able to function, but with reflection I also knew it would not be the right time for me in my journey to take that particular project on. With the current one I am working on, I do feel and have a stronghold on my recovery and have used time management and prioritized things in my life which keep my stress levels down and my abilities are not impaired by lack of judgment due to problematic tigers of symptoms, and I will take this on with heartfelt emotion, and responsibility that I have given towards my recovery and insight into that recovery as well. So reflection allows you to determine with the maturity in recovery of managing it of itself, the ability to allow yourself to succeed in that which you desire to add in your life instead of digress in that which you have attempted or your disease itself.

Again, I cannot stress enough how recovery should be based on the measurable

levels that you put forth for yourself. We are not meant to be robots, and we all

deserve the freedom to make life choices and decisions for ourselves. I do believe

though that one should take on recovery with the prudence of being as successful

as they can in the responsibility of it, without feeling disheartened if the level they

desire is not achieved, or in other words, we can't all become a doctor after a

battle with this disease, and some undue stressors can be left out as long as the

desired quality of live for a consumer is achieved and contentment found.

Chapter 20

Empowerment

What is empowerment? With the fact that you are reading these words or working on a program where this series is utilized, you are practicing empowerment in your choice to participate. You are also practicing empowerment furthermore, not only in the inclusion of your decisions in the process of your own recovery, but also in the realization that through all of the reflection on all of the topics analyzed in this series and your very own formulated measure of success that you have managed through the practice of materials in this series, it is my hope that you have experienced a growth process that will continue throughout your life and in that give you empowerment in every area of your life, not just in the area of mental health recovery. This is the empowerment that those before us that have been caught up in the system, and we ourselves as consumers present have fought long and hard for. We see it in the development of peer support, and now in some clinics' participatory outlining of our own treatment plans, and many other facets that have given us consumers a voice in our own treatment of the disease which we have.

As we as consumers are learning to manage our recovery, we should also be aware of the issues regarding the institutions and organizations which have a heavy influence on the way the treatment of our mental health is unfolded. We do this one for our own sake making sure that we are included in our treatment and the outcomes therein, and two for the greater good of all that are involved in the mental health field whether as consumer, peer provider, or treatment team.

In our growth as consumers it is also necessary for us to show a vigilant stance in advocating for ourselves and others. This also can lead into other areas of our life where we see injustice being done, or change that needs to occur so that people are treated fairly in whatever it is they are involved in or undertaking.

Earlier in this recovery guide series we examined the importance we as consumers had in the inclusion of our care. Not only was it a desire to become well but a responsibility also, to ourselves, or loved ones and society. If we seek to be engaged in our recovery by managing it, using the different tools when we visit our doctors such as the symptom log, or the top ten list when we sit and cooperate with our caseworkers and therapists, we empower ourselves with the ability to become well with the measurements of that success being determined by us as individual consumers.

By starting here by using the concepts of empowerment in our personal journey of recovery, it is hoped that it should transpire to working positively for us in every aspect of our lives, carrying over from that of using it by its conception in our recovery. We will become more involved in all aspects of our lives, which means we are thereby in control of ourselves, our actions, and decisions. We now stand with confidence and the ability to calmly but assertively advocate for ourselves in all the areas that make up who we are as individuals. Part of this advocating for ourselves and others in the system is upholding the standards of parity as put forth by the regulating bodies of the the mental health care authority and, in America, congress itself.

BENEFIT

Perhaps the most enjoyable part of recovery is looking at how we have benefited from our effort in the process. Ensuring that we have kept a belief in our abilities and that we have had an enhancement of our quality of lives is examined. Leaning on the natural resources which are out there in society and immersing ourselves in them as we start to lean on their support, utilizing less and less of the mental health resources as we wean off the system.

We will examine our treatment outcomes; how we consider them to be successful and start to gauge what we want for our future to be. Employment and career potential and guides which assist us in that process as we formulate new roles in society that we wish to fulfill are encouraged.

Also of importance is the way in which we can give back to those who are suffering like we once have, inspiring an end to a stigma which has lasted years upon years and how we can render a change to that problem which all of us as consumers face.

Chapter 21

Belief in One's Self

Believing one's own ability to accomplish anything you put your mind to, or confidence that what you participate in will be done in such a manner where no self doubt is given opportunity to arise, is an all important aspect of recovery for us as consumers. In this portion of the series recovery is motion we have examined three different phases by which we as consumers, utilizing the tools and knowledge gained here, fully grasp a unique and individualized plan of recovery. What is next? The answer is that we not only continue to grow in all aspects of recovery and life, but we begin to benefit from all that we have put in by taking on the responsibility of recovery.

Belief in one's self starts with not only the respect for yourself, but also having others respect who you are as a person; these together make for better self esteem. You begin to become more involved in the natural resources allocated to those in society, without the constant support of mental health clinics of caseworkers, and through participation in those groups or events you make social netting for yourself, and a deeper support network to lean on in times of need.

Respect also means that we respect others for who they are as people. Often times when we are in our stages of illness we want others to conform to who we are, a strange codependency and one which we with the responsibility we have taken on and the proper management of our disease, now take a further look at with the beneficial belief that all may benefit from having ourselves as health members in other peoples life, and society in general. Now it is our turn to allow those in our support system, without a spirit of frustration by us, to heal in the manner that they choose. This healing may mean the release of behavior and episodic times in our own lives when we were symptomatic, and the hurt that they had while going through those times. Respect as we need to see it is a two way street, and that is just the beginning, starting with the deepest support and where it came from when we were in the most need of whoever was there to lend a helping hand or a listening ear.

Working this series we have believed in ourselves the whole way through. We may have had a few speed bumps or even had to take time on more areas and breezed through some of the other topics. Everyone's level of recovery as seen by them is unique and everyone's own level of functioning when coming out of the cold unforgiving world of being mentally ill is different as well, although we as consumers should not judge anyone's pain as less that our own. In doing that we would be left with a series of war stories which would take away from the time needed for recovery and it would most likely also bring isolation from members of the group or peers who by now hopefully you are utilizing.

With our belief that recovery is possible in order, now the belief in ourselves needs to come to fruition which will compliment the two. We may have had that belief the whole way through this series, yet have not examined it thoroughly although it may have been in the back of our minds. What does it mean truly to have belief in ourselves? We know that in recovery it means that we believe that we will overcome the obstacles of symptoms and heal ourselves in the traumas which life had imposed upon us. Translating that towards other life concepts means to believe that we can succeed in other areas as well: employment, if we have been off work for a time, family and relationship and the establishment of those, or reconnection and rebuilding process which sometimes we have to go through. Finding those social supports outside the mental health system as examined earlier will give us not only a new support system where the topic is not only of mental health, where we can enjoy and rest from the worries of our own health, in things such as a bowling league, or golf, softball, or even a band or other arts and crafts that are out there seeking willing participants.

Again as before a top ten list can be used, or the previous one which has been made can be referred to once more allowing time for reflection again and looking at the growth which you have made as an individual enticing more the belief and confidence that you have in yourself, not only as a consumer of services but as an individual with dreams and desires and a person who seeks fulfillment out of life.

What are some tools that can reinforce our own belief in ourselves? A few examples would be in utilizing the outlook of hope, the idea that something can be done. Communication, when you are trying something new, and need a guiding hand, with the ability to utilize its principles you have not only concocted a guiding friend in a new area but an assistant to learn from. Practicing the concepts as we have examined lead to the accomplishment of that which you are trying to achieve, and with the series previous to this one the management of your own personal journey of recovery so that you are in your own eyes a person who has persevered and shown resiliency in overcoming such an obstacle, you have the ability to manage all the tasks in order for you to have confidence in managing other tasks as well.

What also comes along with the believing in yourself is self control and direction over your own life. Not of the life you once led as a victim of a mental disease, but in a life that is new, filled with the possibilities of excitement and rewards. You are now benefiting from all that you have done and the possibilities are out there with the remembrance of what your goals and objectives were to begin with you may pursue those, or as time has gone by, so too do those objectives and goals change and evolve, so with confidence you may evolve with them.

The direction in which you want your life to go is another part of empowerment by which we as consumers, or individuals who have recovered from a disease, now have the ability to choose which way we want our lives to unfold. In terms of employment, relationships, social inclusion, spirituality, and the terms by which we measure as successful engagements, is where we will find that choice and the direction of which to go by.

If you remember early on in this series we examined the thought of how we have a mental disease; the disease does not have us. Here it is no truer to be seen. We have the disease, it does not have us, therefore we are in control to make the choice of which way our lives will go and the direction by which it will take us.

Belief in ourselves means that we have the belief that we can make the proper choices which suit our own needs. There is nothing more important than freedom to choose to do that which you believe, or believe in, nor is it any different than to take that choice away from anyone or anything else. The mental health system has a long history of taking that sacred choice away from us consumers as we have been labeled as insane, crazy, patients, consumers, survivors, and hopefully soon as individuals seeking treatment for a disease. If we choose to give back by advocating for those who are now being inundated to the system, let's do so in such a way that a choice is given to them in regards to their treatment and overall care which they receive. The right to be treated as individuals with dignity, with a disease and all the necessary resources made available for success in functioning while recovering from such an illness.

As I write this portion of belief in oneself and confidence to achieve, I am reminded of a consumer I was helping while a caseworker at a clinic. One of my duties was to travel back and forth to the hospital and transport to the clinic, do an intake and then transport once again to a place of shelter. I was new and was directed to one of the oldest units in the hospital campus on one such outing. I passed by the cemetery, and right next to it was the gerontology psychiatric clinic. I walked through that cemetery and noticed gravesides with no names, some with numbers, and others with years of recent times past. It was a crying heart moment for me as I then walked into the gerontology ward at the hospital, as I knew that the people here had no other place to go, the state psychiatric center was last on the list of where to receive care. I was rushed at with swarms of elderly consumers with questions for me ranging from, am I allowed to go home now, are my children with you, and so forth. It went on until one of the psychiatric nurses eschewed them all away with a mean look on her face and them scared and frightened by her, not wanting to disobey.

I asked for the consumer who I was there to pick up. She then came to the front

and was more than ready to leave. She knew there was nowhere for her to go

but to a boarding home but in my gut I felt as if she desired more than being here

at this facility. She had missed lunch so they gave her something and I knew

where she was going she would not get much more than that for a while. I asked

her if she would like to stop and have a bowl of beans with onions and cheese at

this good eats restaurant in the town which the hospital was located at that I had

found and enjoyed. She was thrilled with having the opportunity to eat good food

and we sat and talked. She told me stories of being in the mental health system

all her life and how her family sent her there years ago when there was nothing to

be done but send her to an asylum as they were called then. When the release of

most patients of psychiatric facilities happened in the seventies she was lucky and

was able to get in at one of the clinics which were rushing to open to fill the void

left by the mass amount of people being released from these hospitals. I gained

so much insight from her, and was sad that even to this day the system had failed

her along the way with her still going in and out of the hospital. She was not on

my caseload and I did not have the opportunity to serve her; how it would have

helped if I did I do not know. What remains is that we have to have the belief and confidence in ourselves, so that we can also have the responsibility to advocate

and bring this feeling of confidence to others still suffering. Let's not make the

final resting place of those lost in the system a small tombstone with their

psychiatric hospital patient number written on it.

We as a unique group of people must have a belief in ourselves that we can

function under any means necessary, symptomatic or not, and the belief that

recovery is best judged by how we see it from our own viewpoint. When we do

that, we then should have the belief that others can recover and that recovery is a

real tangible thing, which does happen, no matter at what age someone is

stricken with mental illness, or at what socio economic status they find

themselves in. To better the system we should have the belief that there are

people who listen to the consumers whom they serve, and truly believe

themselves that recovery is possible. In doing that we can better the likelihood of

our own success, and others now and to come, the statistics I have now are that

90 million Americans now have some form of mental disorder; that is a lot of

people who could not only use our help, but help themselves as well, making

success for all.

Chapter 22

The Enhancement of our

Quality of Life

In parts of this series of topical guides, geared towards igniting the human spirit

towards taking on the work of recovery, we have examined how recovery should

be measured by one's own vision of success and value in the healing which has

occurred within oneself. Quality of life has been a big issue in mental health as

we see that a large number of persons with mental illness rely on the community

mental health system, have become indebted to poor socio economic status, and

focus is often made on needs instead of wants. While making sure someone has

their needs met is important, and wants are pleasant, still that should not be of

the main concern when examining quality of life.

What then is the enhancement of the quality of life? Put simply it is how the

consumer feels about their life as a whole, judging each part in its entirety.

Leaning upon the basic principles which can be found in this recovery is motion series, and using one of the guides most importantly of acceptance. While we examined many areas of what acceptance means to us as consumers and how to apply it in our lives, we should also remember to focus on being content with what we are able to achieve, through overcoming such a debilitating illness.

With this thinking in hand, then what we should strive for is the enhancement of our lives as not only the quality of material things, but the overall enhancement of our lives as individuals. This, through reflection, can be looked at and examined ,and our spirits given even more hope of what may happen for us in life's journey. Not only in the objectives and goals we have achieved, but through the growth we have ascertained as individuals, who upon grasping for the motivation, held on tightly until for that change in our mental health occurred for the better. We then activated our recovery by first accepting that we had a disease which needed to be responsibly handled, communicated to others the traumas and emotional scars which kept us suffering for such a long time, and then began to manage our recovery, being aware of our behavior, nurturing ourselves and our needs in its growth, and taking the time to have pride in the accomplishments we have achieved.

It is my hopes that isolation is not an issue for you at this time or any time throughout. Being involved with people and groups in your life allows you a friendship in which to enjoy your accomplishment if you do so choose to share. If so it is a quality of life issue that should be taken into concern. People together functioning in society make healthy people all around. We examined the relationship issue early on and when it is right or what person should I choose type questions were hard questions which I made an attempt to answer. A romantic type of relationship is one quality of life that many people strive to have, and as a consumer we are more cautious or sometimes not overly cautious enough in that decision.

In viewing what you feel is the enhancement of your own quality of life it is my hopes that you have found some in the recovery process you have underwent in these readings. The department of SAMHA notes that not only should recovery be aimed at achieving a better quality of life for someone who is seeking recovery, but also in their own terms, by their own decisions, and measured by their own values. These are helpful guides in looking at how to reach recovery, but the one who must enhance that quality of life is you the consumer. So I applaud you for all the work you have done thus far and will do in the time to come as you are now benefiting from your hard work.

Quality of life also coincides with the ability for the discontinued use of community service programs by an individual who is using them. This does not mean that you stop seeing a doctor if that is your method of healing, or your alternative way if you have one. What this refers to is that the hope of the community system as a whole, being clinics and hospitals and such, should in essence be to put themselves out of business. Their work is done, or should be done with the idea that they will help heal and find recovery for the individual they are serving. What this means is when you reach the point where you no longer need a caseworker or the state funded system to succeed, then the objective has been reached. There should be a safety net of course as we all know it can take months to get into some of those systems and even years to get disability, and those should be be in place for our benefit against a disease that can sometimes be spontaneous.

What takes its place is community involvement and natural supports with churches, sport activities, organizations where social gatherings occur, or even what we have in place at our different mental health association with trainings and other activities. Statistics have shown that third world countries have a better work retention rate and recovery rate when compared to bigger wealthier countries like the U.S. and U.K. The reason they say that is behind that is that the communities in these countries, although being smaller and better apt to do so, engulf themselves around the individual with a merit of helping them overcome. Here in the U.S. we tend to isolate them even further, enough so that a whole genre of cinema has been created on the subject, most of it dealing with the negative side, giving even more strength to the stigma which we as consumers are forced to live with.

If we are to enhance our quality of living and recover, we should also do the thing that would be prudent and after a time back in the world which once ostracized us, come out of the closet so to speak about our own mental illness and how we were able to overcome it. This would hopefully as we know there are enough of us, although many do not seek treatment, bring about change in a manner that gets people without our disease to say I know him, he is not the crazy type I see in the movies. Also what might help, is that it would give others who have been told they have the disease and live with it suffering in silence the chance to be open and honest about it and seek treatment for it in a open fashion. With these growing numbers, the nay sayers and people who still shy away out of an ignorance of fear, will eventually go away, with the eventual hope of the quality of life we once fought hard for and sought for in change enjoyed by all.

Chapter 23

Natural Resources

and the use of them for mental health consumers

We have examined the use of natural resources and what is meant by them when referring to the term in regards to applying them to mental health needs. It has been my experience I have been able to give guidance to consumers to use them; some I have received poor feedback from and some had nothing but good things to say about it. Again that goes back to choice about how one considers the measure of their quality of life to be. The door of the natural resource is meant to be opened to show that there is a life outside of a revolving outlook of the mental health topic and one which can enrich your life and promote growth. If someone wishes to go by the concept of disability empowerment and be familiar with the different community centers and rec halls as their life, then that is their choice. In remembering that quality of life is an objective to be enhanced, the door is there and someone should be there to open that door and to guide you through it when the time comes if it hasn't already.

With the time constraints on this book I want to go over just a few, for the concept behind it is to examine what each natural resource would bring which would be beneficial to you as the consumer. Whatever your initial motivations were when this journey first began, and whatever they are now if they have evolved, an inward feeling may not be on your top ten list of goals and objectives, could have been so that you can benefit from it in some way.

The first that comes to mind, which are institutions that have been around for a long period of time, are those of fellowshipping with people who belong to a church, synagogue, temple, or what have you. Many of these offer a place to not only practice your spirituality with that of your choice, but much more. They offer companionship in terms of belonging to a specific group, which often helps with people who are still searching for an identity, like many of us as consumers who have lost track of who we are inside, and feel no belonging at times. There are also within this natural resource of a group of fellowshipping believers, charitable causes, some to gain from in times of need where help can be found, and other programs to participate in by way of volunteering. There is much more that you can find here in this good natural resource outside of the realm of mental health system, but in looking at those we can see that just by a few it can be very beneficial.

First off, the spirituality issue is addressed, which we know is essential to one's own recovery in some way or another. Secondly the social inclusion that you will find there where like minded people gather together, putting aside all things of which they have no common ground on, and befriend each other and in support be there for one another on the basis of that spirituality they feel inside as you do yourself. Thirdly, the possibility to participate in kindness found in charitable causes where you can offer your time as a volunteer. There is a great feeling when it comes to being a volunteer, especially if you have been off work for some time and have hopes of going back. It gives you the freedom to work the schedule you want usually as well as having less of a demand on you in terms of being responsible to a boss, a team of employees, or customers. With that, the discussion of employment has yet to come, but will in this series, they are also a good source of networking to find jobs.

There are sporting and game leagues which you can participate in, or even personal exercise routines which will bring not only a holistic approach to your recovery healing the mind and body, but also bringing entertainment and companionship. Becoming involved in a sporting league in particular can bring confidence as you see your sporting game improve, companionship with one another on the team, and a healthy regular rate of exercise for the body. Personal exercise routines will challenge you to keep yourself in shape and fit, and can bring along with that an improvement of self esteem with loss of weight and muscular formation from working out.

Belonging to some type of arts group would also be a natural resource to involve yourself in if that is your cup of tea. Some are even spiritual in nature, giving yourself the opportunity to write poems that may be used in some form of meditation by yourself. They bring about feelings of accomplishment, as you see whatever it is that you decide to participate in come to fruition. Along with that will also come the camaraderie of being with a group which promotes good social functioning.

Within all of these, and more natural resources, you will also find respect. You will find that people respect you for who you are and what you bring to the table and you in turn will find that respecting others' input and participation in your life will motivate you to stay involved in your recovery. Respect is a precious thing and must go both ways, to an individual and from another individual for it to work successfully.

For me in my recovery I found the most holistic part of my recovery in the natural resources which I choose to participate in. I made, yes, a list again, of things I enjoyed, or remember enjoying before the onset of the mental illness and loss of interest in things. I decided to start off slow and it was hard sometimes to get motivated to do some of the things that I enjoyed doing, like lifting weights and working out, being that I had let my body get so physically out of shape it was hard to get back into it. But the people I met at the gym kept me motivated, and I even met someone who worked out the same time as I did that was having problems with his own son. He was very worried about what his son was going through, which was much akin to what I had gone through early on in my life. With the drugs, and gang affiliations, his son was also diagnosed with a mental disorder, his last time being sent to the youth authority. So in my efforts to keep myself involved in a holistic approach as a part of my recovery, and using the resource of a small gym, I was also able to give support and answers as well as a listening ear to someone who needed it at the time.

I also tied an arts and crafts hobby into my life one year at Christmas time, when I purchased a train set for my son. He was amazed and I actually found out from his mother that it was one of the things that he had asked Santa for, but I was unaware of that, I just wanted to not only get involved with something that both my son at the age of six and I could do and be special as an indoor activity. The train was the answer to that search. It turned in to a behavior modification tool as well, when I told him that we would purchase more pieces for him. As time went on I found out that he was getting better reports from his teachers on proper behavior in class. I during this time was truly benefiting from my recovery efforts. Not only that, but I could see the benefits without having to delve deep through the dark lenses of the illness to catch a glimpse; they were protruding right out in front of me. This will come with time when you truly take on the responsibility of recovery and work it in a way that conforms to your own personal style. You will be thankful that you took on that responsibility as you reap the rewards of your hard work. You will see that it will not only be beneficial to you, but to those all around you who love and care about you.

Chapter 24

Employment and Career Outlook

I spent over two years as a job coach, job developer, and employment specialist, while also taking a course where I earned my undergraduate certificate in supported employment. I had the privilege to serve many, ranging from all types of what are known and labeled as disabilities. I did not see a disability, what I saw was an ability needing to be pronounced, which they already had inside themselves. That is how we should look at ourselves sometimes, as people with many abilities inside, that upon benefiting from our recovery actions will be more pronounced and people will take a closer look at who we are as a unique group of resilient people.

It can sometimes be a scary decision for a consumer. When should I go to work, am I ready for work, am I going to lose my benefits, these are all questions that we ask ourselves when approaching that time. All of these are confusing items to be ironed out, and the government in America tried with different campaigns like the ticket to work and so forth, which in my opinion, frankly was more out to help the tax payer and the fed rather than the sufferer of a illness or condition which made work either unable to participate in, or scarcely able to do from time to time.

The supported employment programs have come along way in America from their first use, during the world wars when men coming home from battle with wounds and limitations needed a system to allow these men to get back to the jobs they left in order to go protect our freedoms. Congress saw that and more when they developed the ADA, and included in that were all people whose right to work was limited due to some reason or another. It has even come an even longer way since I entered the workforce and began as a job coach over nine years ago. The rules have changed, the billing has changed, and all mostly to benefit the consumer who is receiving services, making sure that the vendor providing those services does the job of acquiring a position of gainful employment with opportunity for advancement.

Yet for some reason, although many mental health consumers are getting needed help from state agencies like DARS, it can sometimes feel that a consumer must jump through hoops in order to be able to get permission for their services to be rendered to them as disabled Americans. This first came to light for me when I was working at a non profit organization as the director of peer supported employment. It was a great idea and one backed by the state on two levels, whereby we used job coaches and sometimes even developers whose prior requirement was to be a peer support specialist. We had some success but the unfortunate chain of events they call cutbacks, which usually means cutting back on mental health services mostly in the states budget, eventually forced the non profit to close its doors.

While at the non profit, I found out that in order for a person with a disability of mental illness to be green lighted for services, they had to first take several tests to see if they were ready to go to work. I am fond of assessments as they are a good tool, but not when it comes to the say so if a man or woman has the right to try and work in this country under an act by congress which should allow them the assistance if they needed it. What this left was me having to answer many questions coming from people whom I served on the ACT team at one of my other positions who were familiar with me and wanted my assistance in finding work. Again another time I felt I had let down one of my peers and had to side with the bureaucracy of a doctor being able to make the decision on whether or not someone is suitable for work. What edged me on about this so much was that a year prior to that I had attended a workshop where the speaker Ed Knight was there and had much to say about the concept of working with a mental disability. The portion which spoke out to me the most is that you do not have to be symptom free in order to work. That was it, it is a persons choice to work, and without the chance they will never slowly get acclimated back into it.

The second reason I feel that not enough is given into getting a mental health consumer back into work, from the standpoint of an organization, is that they now have a special program especially for consumers with mental illness. This special program consists of bouncing the person around month to month for a period of time to see if they can get use to working. I understand the concept of allowing time for someone who may or may not have a strong history of work experience get the feel for daily life as an employee, but there are other things that I feel are more important to consider.

In doing it with this methodology, you instill firstly the idea that hopping from one job to the next is OK and expected. Two, they never get a feel for what they are really doing and learning at the place they are in one month's time. Three, in doing it like this it never gives the consumer the opportunity for advancement, promotion, pay rise, or even a regularly set schedule.

I am by no means trying to scare you away from the working environment or the programs out there that seek to do good for consumers with the intentions they have, and here is where you need to be your best advocate for yourself. Part of SAMHSA has within its list we examined that recovery also means the ability to be in control over one's own life. So as you venture into this world of work do so with confidence in yourself, the knowledge of what is before you, and maybe some tricks of the trade I can give you on how to get that position you really desire.

First and foremost know now that the position that the helping resources are taking now on securing employment for someone with a disability is that of choice of the consumer, which must have opportunity for advancement and livable wages. With that in mind don't let yourself be put off by a vendor who forces what those in the business call the three f's, fast food, flowers, and fun, meaning that you either have only the opportunity to work at a fast food chain, water flowers in a department store, or work at a amusement park. While these are not detestable jobs and the people who do them are not below anyone's level, vendors do tend to center in on the jobs which have no means of advancement opportunity, and are often seasonal, all because they are easy to find placement in.

Be an advocate for yourself as well. If a vendor has a job lined up for you and you do not want it then let them know, but also be reasonable as unemployment rates vary from time to time in areas. In advocating for yourself take on the responsibility of managing your time allotted for your own input and work required to find that position. You can do job searches on your own and work in tandem with the vendor so that a good resolution to your desire of becoming gainfully employed will come to fruition.

Lastly as mental health consumers, we know from our experiences that often times we have periods of job interruption where no work was done. In building resumes and such there are ways to show that you progressed in learning and still have that ability to do a job when sometimes the absence of employment on your resume may look not so good to an employer. One good detail is to put in a period of time when you were ill that you were taking care of a family member who was ill, after all it is the truth you were ill and you were taking care of yourself.

Working of itself is such a fruitful experience for us as consumers. It gives us social opportunities with co-workers that can enhance our lives. Working also gives us the ability to achieve a better quality of life, not only with our needs and wants being met financially, but through the feelings of being needed in life and accomplishing something on a daily basis. Having more responsibility, and managing that responsibility once it is in motion, is a very beneficial thing.

Chapter 25

Formulation of Roles

We all have roles in our life to fulfill, and with the disease of mental illness sometimes those roles are lost among us, forgetting who we once were in recovery, and others are harmed at times such as our roles in relationships and societal obligations. As consumers it is helpful to iron out these roles, to see where they need mending and to see where we need to place them back into our lives. Having a role in life such as a parent, a brother, a partner or friend, can be rewarding when it is responsibly managed and nurtured by the way of understanding, giving, sharing, and many other fruits which come from being involved as a participant in life's roles.

One of our roles which we can't overlook is the role of being a mental health consumer or survivor. Although this may not be a role which we have chosen outright, it is one that we are somewhat forced to fulfill. In fulfilling that role we do so with the hope that we will as our peers have through perseverance, show the resiliency that we have as a unique group to overcome the troublesome aspects of the disease itself. We do this leaning upon our strengths, and leaning upon one another growing with group feedback as we engage in our recovery with others in support groups and the like.

In all actuality, it can be said that one of the motivators which we have for being engaged in recovery is the restoration or roles which we once had in our lives, ones which we succeeded in with responsibility towards them, and harm not being done to them by the mental illness and behavior which sometimes showed injury to them. This is where we realize that when relating to our support systems we should with due diligence work together knowing that those who support and care about us have feelings and emotions too, some of which are caused by fighting alongside us this disease of mental illness. Knowing that it has an effect on them as well, and taking the opportunity to show thankfulness and care toward their hurt is truly a growth point in our recovery where by we can establish these roles in a healthy manner.

As a mental health consumer/survivor, I realize the importance of having a strong support system. Support systems can include a significant other, family members, friends, and even other mental health consumers. Chances for recovery are greatly improved when we are able to lean on a strong support system. Our support system gives us encouragement and understanding. A support system is there for us during times of accomplishment and troublesome times as well. A support system allows us to let someone assist us or take over everyday tasks that we might not be able to do at certain times during our recovery, from simple things such as running an errand to more complex tasks such as managing finances. We hope that our support system understands what we are going through and, just as important, we need to be aware of the commitment our support system is making in being there for us. They fight alongside us in the goal of defeating the disease, helping us to live a more fruitful life as we manage the symptoms of our illness.

It comforts us when we know that our supporters have understanding of what we are going through. This involves understanding not only our symptoms but also our dreams and aspirations we have as individuals. We all want that "American Dream," just as any other person does. To have the feeling of being needed and respected for who we are, and the contributions that we are able to give to society, give us a sense of being more than mere outcasts. Sometimes we feel that we have a lack of freedom, literally such as when we are hospitalized, as well as at other times, such as when making life choices. Oftentimes we feel like a captive to the medication that we take. Some of us question what it would be like to not take medications at all, especially when we fellow ex-patients are no longer taking medications. We often feel stressed when, at times, we are forced to depend on government programs, hoping that they will keep us afloat. Many of us who are parents struggle with the stress of being able to provide for our family and children, just like other parents who do not suffer from what we generically call a mental illness. The above are just a few of the many situational stressors that we feel impact us on a greater level than those who are not going through recovery. We want to know that our loved ones understand.

Even though at times we may feel overwhelmed by the stressors in our lives, we as consumers/survivors should also have a respect and an admiration for our supporters who see us experiencing them and empathize with us as we continue on our journey toward recovery. Just like we are aware of our own emotional upheavals, we should have an empathetic understanding of the individuals in our support system.

Family mental health counselors and coalitions such as NAMI also support us by bringing our fight into the public array, acting as a rallying cry for better care and up to date recovery techniques. We as consumers need to also take a stance for ourselves and show the appreciation that we have for those who are supporting us.

At times when we have feelings of being controlled by our support system. We may be inclined to disregard their advice. At these times, we just need to be mindful that they are looking out for our best interest and take the advice for what it is, advice of a caring supporter. Our support system suffers alongside us, not in the symptoms themselves, but rather as an emotionally involved person who sees the pain and obstacles that we deal with and how it affects us. We need to reach to them and show appreciation for their decision to stay with us.

In working in the mental health field as a caseworker, I have seen individuals who have a strong support network consisting of family and close friends. I have also seen individuals whose network consists only of those people who are paid to be there, such as doctors, therapists and social workers. Those of us who have a strong network of supporters in our everyday lives need to take time to be thankful and appreciative. As for those of us who may have alienated the individuals who we once leaned upon for support, it is my hope that our doctors, therapists and social workers can help us learn to re-connect with those individuals and help us fill empty spaces with new supporters and help us to re-establish those supports we once had. When we gain a better understanding of how each of us has been affected by this terrible disease, we have a greater chance in recovering from it together.

Of course there are many other roles which we as consumers restore to ourselves in everyday life. Roles as students that could take us further into a goal of what we wish to accomplish and make a purpose in life. As we have gone through this transformation, the personal individual choices you have made while utilizing these series, you have most likely engaged back into the world formulating roles which you fill in life by going through the topics and putting into practice the recovery therein. So upon using reflection gain a sense once again of the growth you have made within yourself by putting your motion into recovery, acting on it, managing it, and now finally seeing the benefits.

I was speaking with a peer one day and he was in what I like to call the doldrums, feeling down and unsure of himself, so I asked him what was bothering him. He told me that he didn't see any changes in his life. I then asked him so I understand that you want changes in your life. He confirmed that that was what he had said and I asked him if he had done anything to make changes happen to look at what he had going on in his life now. He went through several things such as activities he was involved in, groups he participated in, and then it hit him, he was so caught up with still trying to discover who he was that he wasn't able to see that what he was doing was who he was, that he had been in the process of making something of himself. It is funny that oftentimes when we are really engaging in life we tend to overlook our accomplishments because we are so busy not living in the moment with them. We have a one track mind of sorts which sometimes tends to keep us focused on the question of whether we are doing enough. Instead it is often a healthy thing to participate in our lives with the things that we do by learning to engage our whole selves in whatever it is that we participate in. It's like the old saying says, take time to smell the flowers, and not only that, while your garden grows manage it with care and benefit from everything that it produces.

Chapter 26

Inspiring an End To Stigma

The idea of stigma as it relates to mental health consumers has been around for a long time. It is embellished in Hollywood, selling the rare cases that make up about one percent of us people who are labeled as crazy, or insane. In some cases families are embarrassed to speak about it if a family member has come down with a mental illness. Our transportation system is wary about people who might be bi polar or suffer from schizophrenia as they have seen rare episodes of displays of anxiety and panic happen while traveling. All in all these are some of the many reasons and displays of stigma that exist today, which we as consumers are forced to deal with and try to change.

This changing will not occur overnight, although there would be a possibility that it could. As we noted that in third world countries the community gathers around the person who is stricken with a mental illness, engaging them in every activity and keeping them away from the ruins of isolation. They accept when the symptoms do occur and adjust to meet the needs of the person the community has a vested interest in.

If our fast paced capitalistic world of me first were to practice what is been done successfully by third world countries, whose level of income prevents medication and information on the illness to reach them, I ask myself what would occur. I have come to the realization that my country, the U.S., has statistics of mental illness being at 90 million people; that is quite a lot. Many of course keep it to themselves and are able to hide it and do not seek treatment, or if they do it is in a private setting and kept separate from other facets of their lives.

What were to happen if all of these people came out of the closet so to speak, and told their friends, their family members, and others in their life that they had a mental illness? Would these people in their life be surprised, or would they suggest that they knew all along? Whatever the outcome, a stigma is best fought in a large group withstanding those who have prior beliefs and then displaying that those beliefs are far from the average. Tom in accounting is bi polar one might say, I never knew that, he seems like a normal guy. After that initial reaction and more coming forward then mental illness wouldn't seem so dark and debilitating as it is displayed or sometimes is without proper treatment.

Our part as consumers who live the life of a consumer out in the open, do have the choice to keep things private. However isn't it a responsibility to give back to the part of society which helped you recover from a mental illness? If that is the case then we are all grooming ourselves into being leaders of a field that once for treatment took a large nail and hammered it into our head hoping it would quell voices; oh, how far we have come. Yet we have so much further to go towards ending not only stigma but seeking out for better treatments in stabilization, more rights for choices of treatment, and parity in care when compared to that of physical medicine.

So what is it that we can do as consumers who have chosen the life of recovery? We can act as an advocate, join our local organizations which with their strength in numbers have the power to create change. We are a resilient people, unique in that we have found the strength to overcome the power and control which the mind can have upon a person. We thus have a lot to give with ideas which can be written and shared, and through our activities such as art promote change in the structures of Hollywood and the media showing that people with a mental health issue are more people to be looked up at as people of strength with great heroism to overcome adversity, instead of the guy down the hall talking to you with intent to harm.

Let us inspire an end to stigma by maintaining our recovery, consistently engaged in it, and if someone asks tell them I have overcome, I am now living life with many more attributes. Relish in the good times in life, let your family members and friends see you out and about making memories, this news will spread. If you seek out a romantic relationship and you feel the time is ready to discuss health issues, start with one of the positive movies that are out there that inspire hope and courage among those of us who have battled and claimed victory over this generic disease we call mental illness.

Chapter 27

Treatment Outcomes

In looking at treatment outcomes the first point which comes to mind is from that

of a clinical standpoint meeting the check marks of being symptom free,

functioning, and involved in society as well as many other clinical points. It's

funny to think how when we as consumers are in the process of having our

treatment guide planned for us, often times we are left out of the equation and

no input from us is asked. This is funny because we are the ones who are

hopefully making this treatment become successful. In recent years consumers have had more input in regards to our treatment and it is my hope that this trend continues.

One of the reasons I took on writing this book, hopefully after the initiation of these recovery principles helping people, was to be able to put it into the format of a workbook. The study that I will refer to is the pillars of peer support by which it suggest ways in which we as consumers can be involved in our own treatment and it follows itself up with another study showing over a certain period of time how the input of consumer involvement and having a peer support personnel on a treatment team affect recovery. This was done by comparing it with another clinic which had no peer support. The study found that while there was a better satisfaction in customer service done so by the ones with a peer on board, a peer on board the team still showed the same results in regards to recovery.

While I don't know all about this particular study, I do ask myself what is it that we define recovery by. This book is meant to lead and guide a person on the path of recovery but more to give knowledge which they can implement and format into their own lives as every individual's idea of recovery is different. That is the basis of being non linear; a different set of measures of recovery, looking at it by how the consumer sees recovery taking place in their life, and that is what I hoped that this book would do for my fellow peers. To give them the foundations by which I have gained my recovery and all the knowledge I have through my education, experience in the field, and more importantly being a consumer for over 14 years.

Treatment outcomes can be divided as the clinics do into different phases and tie lines, and since money does play an important role in having resources for recovery there does have to be a basis by which treatment outcomes can be determined. Clinics should be in the business of putting themselves out of business, meaning that they want to find a way to heal mental illness so that as others come in many others are leaving and living life with the quality which they have found and are happy with.

I am not a radical who says rebuild the whole system, that is why you see many mainstream recovery topics and clinical practices in this book. I do believe however that recovery as it is redefined should also have a redefinition about how it is processed and taken place by the therapeutic teams who serve us. This is my look at recovery, and one which has helped me stay engaged. I hope that it has assisted you in your own journey and that you feel inspired to pass it on to friends and get it in the hands of people at clinics and others who make decisions about what we as individuals recovering from a mental disease need and want as far as topics discussions, practices, and most importantly keeping recovery in motion.

www.ingramcontent.com/pod-product-compliance
Lightning Source LLC
Chambersburg PA
CBHW030618220526
45463CB00004B/1336